sleep
recovery

The five step
yoga solution to
restore your rest

sleep
recovery

LISA SANFILIPPO

GREEN TREE
LONDON • OXFORD • NEW YORK • NEW DELHI • SYDNEY

GREEN TREE
Bloomsbury Publishing Plc
50 Bedford Square, London, WC1B 3DP, UK

BLOOMSBURY, GREEN TREE and the Green Tree logo are
trademarks of Bloomsbury Publishing Plc

First published in Great Britain 2020

A catalogue record for this book is available from the British Library

Library of Congress Cataloguing-in-Publication data has been applied for

ISBN: TPB: 978-1-4729-5631-6; eBook: 978-1-4729-5630-9

2 4 6 8 10 9 7 5 3 1

Typeset in Gentium Basic by Austin Taylor
Printed and bound in the UK by CPI Group (UK) Ltd. Croydon, CR0 4YY

To find out more about our authors and books visit www.bloomsbury.com
and sign up for our newsletters

Contents

....

INTRODUCTION TO SLEEP RECOVERY

Waking up happy starts now

WE ALL KNOW A MAGICAL UNICORN SLEEPER: lucky people who can do *whatever they want*, put their bodies in bed at any hour, close their eyes, and wake up eight hours later with no problem, feeling totally refreshed. I'm not one of those people. I have to take care with what I do all day for my sleep to stay in tune. And even if *you* were once such a magical beast with easy, carefree sleep, I'm guessing this isn't the case for you right now – so what we will do together in this book is uncover *simple things* you can do for yourself, any time, anywhere, to ensure you get the good-quality sleep you need so you wake up refreshed, with plenty of energy for the day ahead. You'll never have to worry about your sleep again.

For many years now, I've been holding workshops that gather people together to sort out what's going on, and to help them find lasting sleep *solutions*. If you were there, I'd ask you to raise your hand when I get to the problem(s) you recognise:

+ Are you struggling to fall asleep, even though you're exhausted?
+ Are you waking up in the middle of the night with your mind – or your heart – racing?

- Are you waking up after only a few hours' sleep and feeling like the day drags on in a fog?
- Do you seem to sleep forever and still not feel rested?
- Are you here because you want to help your partner, your child, or a friend who's having trouble sleeping?

By raising your hand and looking around, you'd see how many other people in the room share your problem with sleep. Then I'd tell you that I too had most of those problems, and wish I'd known that I wasn't alone. I've had nearly every kind of sleepless night and all manner of insomnia, but I've learned to repair my sleep and manage my energy all day – and because of this, I *know* I can help you find *your* way through it.

Insomnia and me

As a long-suffering insomniac, I bought every lotion and potion, tried every technique, tool and prop, every herbal remedy, aromatherapy, and pillow spray: you name it, I tried it. These *all* failed to get to the root of the problem. What I came to understand is that sleeplessness is a symptom of *something else* in our lives that has gone out of balance.

During a bout of devastating night-after-night insomnia in my mid-twenties, I visited my doctor in desperation. She checked me over and found nothing wrong with my breathing, my thyroid or my hormones: there was nothing *physically* wrong with me that would cause insomnia. She then gave me a great gift by refusing to prescribe sleeping pills; since I was so young, she worried that she'd be encouraging a lifetime of dependency. This was a good call on her part: I *had* to find a non-drug way to get to sleep and stay asleep. She suggested that I start doing yoga, and work with a counsellor or therapist. What she could see – but didn't articulate in so many words – was that my sleep problems had multiple roots, in my body and mind: my psychology, my nervous system, my emotions and maybe something deeper still.

I decided that if I didn't do something about my sleeplessness and the chaos it caused me, I'd be in for a life sentence. Out of desperation, and because I really wasn't willing to tolerate a lifetime of crippling exhaustion, I took her advice – and in the process became a yoga therapist and psychotherapist myself.

How I learned to 'just relax'

Back when I was at my lowest ebb, if you'd told me to 'just relax' I'd probably have wanted to shout at you: 'I AM TRYING TO RELAX!' If I could, I really would have, but I genuinely didn't know *how*. Life involved perpetual low-level tension, some part of which would never budge. Times that were supposed to be fun (senior prom, graduation day, birthdays, vacations, at the hairdresser, even in a massage) were not: on edge the whole time, the knot in my stomach was a constant. The sense of tightness and its companion, anxiety, got worse when I'd try to sleep. I'd get into bed, slowing down for the first time all day, and notice the buzzing in my legs, shoulders bunched up to my ears, brow permanently furrowed – even my *feet* felt tight.

My first yoga class came free with my membership to a gym occupying a converted bank in Brooklyn. The basement cardio studio, free weights occasionally crashing into the floor overhead, was yoga-fied with foil-wrapped tea lights around the perimeter of the room. As the grey-haired yoga teacher, clad in floaty linen, offered each *maddeningly* slow stretch, I held back the urge to bolt from the room. But her voice was firm and soothing and her poetic suggestions held my interest. 'Lift your arms and *ribbon* your breath up your spine.' 'Okay,' I thought, 'I'll play'. I bent, and I breathed.

About half an hour into the class, we did this *twisting thing*. The teacher described its action 'like wringing out a wet towel' and when I wrung, a disturbing pain shot through my chest and back. Unravelling from the position, I felt something else, the *opposite* of pain – a tingly feeling in my ribs. The knot in my stomach felt smaller and one of my shoulders sank *lower* than the other. Interested, I gave in to the idea of seeing the class through to the end. In the locker room mirror afterwards, my eyes looked *bigger* than usual, the creases in my forehead softened. My lungs seemed to take in more air and my customary fast stomp home was more of a saunter, like floating on a cushiony pair of sneakers.

What I know now is that a deep stretch, paired with smooth, even breathing, gets the muscle fibres to unstick themselves, and knots in the muscles, called adhesions, can begin to unravel. It can feel like something is being torn apart, because that's exactly what's happening. When I stretched areas of my body that I'd never felt before, I became aware of places I'd never related to until then. The space and openness, the increase in circulation and the relaxation that came from it made the discomfort and the oddity of it worth it, and I've come to associate that sensation with deeply pleasant *softening* and *clarifying*.

These days, I do yoga as if I were tidying a room: opening up the cupboards and cleaning out even the places I couldn't initially see. It's a lot like the way the Japanese tidying guru Marie Kondo suggests we declutter: whisk everything into the centre of the room – clothes out of the drawers, turn out the closets, empty the laundry baskets and get all the boxes out from underneath the bed, see it all together to become aware of what's really there – and then make choices. Throw stuff away, or put it back in a more organised way.

The yoga stretches bring different parts of your body into focus. Feeling all the little creaks and tweaks from *every part* means I stop squirrelling tension away in hidden cupboards and corners in my body. This stretching consciously with breath is a clear-out – not turning a power hose to the place, when a fine feather duster will do the work. The practice I do, and which I offer you in this book, is subtle and kind. I find it pleasant enough to *seduce* me into doing it, rather than it feeling like an obligation, simultaneously calming but strong. Doing the pre-sleep yoga stretches cleans the gunk out of my body so that it's clear and spacious – ready for good rest.

The sleeplessness epidemic

During the height of my insomnia, I was convinced I was the only one awake in the middle of the night, thrashing around in the sheets, my limbs twitching. I now know it wasn't just me and that, since then, the global problem has become a whole lot worse: perhaps we've even reached a 'sleeplessness epidemic'. Today, in many Western post-industrial countries, including my native United States and my now-home in the UK, *up to 20 per cent* of the adult population has clinically diagnosable insomnia, meaning that one in five of us meets the clinical definition: because of our sleep problems, we are significantly impaired – that is, more than three times per week for more than three months at a time – in our day-to-day ability to function. And even greater numbers of us are simply *unsatisfied* with our sleep or *worried* about it.

I've seen insomnia and sleep problems go from something suffered in silence to a common complaint; and it seems that, as a society, we have become *obsessed* with sleep. Not a day goes by when I don't see a new sleep-related product advertised or a new article in a broadsheet, tabloid or social media post offering 'top sleep tips'. It's not surprising: we've spent nearly a generation thinking sleep was something negotiable – and quotes like 'I'll sleep when I'm dead' and 'Sleep is for wimps' have been thrown about by everyone from rock stars to politicians.

A recent wave of books now highlights how *important* sleep is to our well-being on every level. It seems strange to me that we would need to read these books – almost like saying 'eating is important'. But then again, in our culture, the basics have become problematic.

As we have become alienated from our bodily, creaturely selves, the very things we rely on for our survival – eating and sleeping – have become deeply disordered for so many of us. Another creaturely urge – sex – seems similarly problematic, with people feeling alienated or over-indulging in unhealthy ways in record numbers. You may argue with me, but I believe that when done well and in a healthy way, getting good and nourishing sleep, like sex, involves intimacy, safety and awareness. So, recovering our sleep restores trust, tenderness, and sensitivity to our bodies and to every aspect of ourselves: body, energy, mind, emotions and spirit. This book gives you a map to find your way back to a connection with your creaturely self.

A cue that change is needed

If you can't sleep, you may have some of the same thoughts and feelings I did when in the depths of my sleep-deprived desperation:

I can't let go.

I can't *stop*.

I can't trust.

I just need to get this next thing done.

Something isn't right.

I can't even remember how it feels to rest.

Something keeps waking me up.

The fundamental key to Sleep Recovery, which underpins every step in this process, is that when some part of ourselves is out of balance, we get cues that say 'change is needed'. These cues may start as whispers, then become exclamations, and if you don't listen, then finally your whole system is shouting at you. While for some people the whispers and shouts come through in the form of digestive problems, skin breakouts or other health problems, for me – and for the people I describe in this book – sleeplessness is the message that something is wrong. It's like the 'canary in the coal mine' telling us that something isn't right, that change is needed.

If, like I was, you are miserable enough, or are tired of feeling less than your best, you too will be motivated to make changes to restore your sleep – and you don't need to spend years putting the pieces together. I've laid it out for you. The approach I offer is the result of over 20 years' research into medical, psychological, traditional and even some very non-traditional approaches – and while the programme is yoga-based, there is nothing woo-woo about it; you won't have to become a contortionist, change religion or join a cult! I have simply brought together the most useful parts of all these disciplines, which, together with my own experiences of sleeplessness, my training and clinical work as a yoga therapist and psychotherapist, and my work with hundreds of people, along with a little trial and error, have contributed to the creation of this five-step guide. *Sleep Recovery* gives you the knowledge, tools and resources to repair your own natural ability to rest, starting tonight, and will enable you to do this for the rest of your life.

The tools and practices in this book are ones I've used for years, and I've seen them change people on every level. I'm not an expert in all things sleep now as a career choice, or because it seemed interesting academically. The things I've learned and offer you here have been my lifelines. The tools have helped me to repair my body, mind and emotional responses, the most elemental parts of my life, and sharing them with other people feels meaningful and soulful. It's this sense of purpose that I see many of my clients have lost, and part of the waking-up process that sleeplessness can nudge us into is about just that – meaning, value and a sense of purpose.

I no longer *worry* about my sleep, and I generally have plenty of energy – because I use the meditation or restorative practices during the day if I need them. These aren't just things I do for my sleep, but practices of nourishing myself through body, energy, mind, heart and soul. What I'm offering you as practices for sleep recovery are actually tools for awakening – for feeling a sense of wellness, spiritedness and joy. I will help you get to the root of your sleep problems, and if you follow the five steps described and do the practices along the way, you'll sleep more, rest more deeply and wake up, on the whole, happier and healthier.

How to use the five-step programme

In each step in this programme, you'll get new information and tools to repair the places where your sleep has broken. When I teach group classes, I spend one week on each of the steps. Reading the whole book once and then doing a step each week is a great way to maintain momentum and see results. You can, of course, spend more time with each step. Start at the chapter that grabs your attention most and adapt as you need. But remember – it only works if you are willing to take action, make changes, and put what you learn into practice.

The five steps of sleep recovery

Step 1	**Repair your body**
	• Learn the Basic Yoga Breath.
	• Practise the Simple Sleep Sequence.
	• Learn how the physiology of sleep works in order to stop sabotaging your sleep.

Step 2	**Repair your energy**
	• Make your nervous system less nervous: Learn how your nervous system works and how your breathing and the ways you use your energy will help you to recover your sleep.
	• Change how you breathe for sustainable energy and to prepare for sleep.
	• Learn to 'put energy back on the grid' during the day with rest postures.

Step 3	**Reclaim your mind**
	• Learn about the brainwave patterns involved in sleep and how to repair your ability to get to sleep and stay asleep using simple practices.
	• Un-busy your mind, manage your thoughts, and retrain your brain to sleep better.
	• Use the Captain's Log/journal, mindfulness tools and easy-to-learn meditation techniques.

Step 4	**Restore a sense of calm**
	• Get to the heart of your sleep problems, looking at how you deal with the emotional aspect of sleepless nights.
	• Learn how the effects of trauma can change your sleep and how to recover from post-traumatic sleep problems.
	• Learn a simple emotional release technique that can help you to sleep better at night.

Step 5	**Release fear, reawaken happy**
	• Look at soulful ways to *wake up* happier for the rest of your life, using your sleeplessness as a wake-up call.

SLEEP RECOVERY

A new approach

I LISTEN TO THE COMPLAINTS of people who come to sleep-related workshops, and most often they say something like 'I can't switch off'. If you want to recover your sleep, let's agree on one thing first: you are not a machine. A vital part of restoring your sleep is working *with* your very creaturely, human nature.

In this programme, you will reconnect to your human nature. To start with, we don't like pain and we avoid discomfort. This means that we can run ourselves ragged, propping ourselves up with everything from caffeine to cocaine, sugar to shopping as ways to fill our time, to make ourselves feel good, or feel better. We are largely overstimulated. Most of us who have trouble sleeping sidestep the discomfort of tiredness during the day by drinking caffeine or mentally charging up in ways that stimulate our internal stress response so that we can push through, rather than simply resting. There's a lot of social pressure to do this, and our workplaces may seem to demand it. But most people I meet demand more of themselves than is actually required by their home or work life. Not wanting or being able to stop, or to let go, is a bad habit – and it's killing our sleep.

And even worse, the siren call of scrolling, clicking, flicking and swiping can lead to hours of reading, watching, learning, porning, messaging, social-media-ing, shopping or anything else you can do connected to a screen. If this happens to you, you're not the only one. Maintaining a highly stimulated state and seeking to overcome our discomfort in ways that don't actually nourish us can do us more harm than good.

This, according to the latest evidence, goes back to the way we were taught to deal with stress as small children. Our Western culture does not teach us to follow our innate body sense, nor to discharge strong emotions or physical tension, so we have not really learned to identify and listen to what we need to nourish ourselves. If we have sleep problems, we may not be so skilled at effectively self-soothing, relaxing and resting. In a very real and vital sense, recovering our sleep is about acting like a good parent putting a baby to bed, but doing this for ourselves by creating feelings of safety, soothing and calming, setting in place good habits, and helping the most vulnerable part of ourselves feel safe enough to let go.

Stop comparing ... and stop despairing

Not only are you a human being, you are a unique combination of physical, mental, emotional and even spiritual tendencies and capacities. While we all want to know what's 'normal', there is a huge variety in what's healthy from person to person, based on our physical makeup and our emotional/psychological character. You may compare your sleep to an *ideal* and find yourself lacking, which will make you more stressed and worried, further undermining your ability to sleep. You may expect to work the same hours or have the same leisure time as others, and this can make you crazy. You may even compare yourself to how things were for you at another stage of your own life, or think you need to have the same abilities – and the same sleep – as your partner or friends. There is a slogan used in addiction recovery circles that applies really well to sleep: **'Compare ... and despair!'** Through this book, you'll track your sleep so you know what's really happening (page 24–25) and you'll do simple, effective practices that change how you feel and how you sleep. Each one is backed up by evidence and also by the experiences of other people, in whose stories you may recognise something of yourself. You'll find your Sleep Type, put in place good habits, relearn how to rest on every level and find *your* best pathway to Sleep Recovery.

What makes Sleep Recovery different?

So, how is Sleep Recovery different from other approaches you might have tried? In restoring the connection to our human nature, Sleep Recovery replaces our most damaging and self-sabotaging habits with more helpful skills and tools that are integrated with how you live, in both subtle and profound ways. This is different from many contemporary methods of overcoming sleep problems, which generally take one of three main approaches, each offering important pieces of the puzzle while missing out other, vital, pieces. You may have already heard of or used some of these methods.

1 **Chemical fixes** can include anything that changes your state through ingesting something: sleeping pills prescribed by a doctor or found over the counter, supplements you find through a nutritionist or decide to take yourself, or special diets or supplementation.

2 **Daily habits**, called 'sleep hygiene', including wake and sleep times, minimising night-time blue-light exposure, and managing your sleep environment.

3 **Mind-over-matter techniques**, including cognitive-behavioural approaches, that tell you not to worry about sleep and to manage your perceptions around it – from counting sheep to using other, more complicated mind-relaxing tools.

While they all have something of value, if your sleep has been broken there's an essential piece (or pieces) I'll bet you're missing. I'll give you a way to sleuth out your most valuable keys to sleeping better, using the Sleep Tracker and the Five Steps to Sleep Recovery.

The Five Steps: A map

The Sleep Recovery Map shows you the essential elements you need to restore healthy sleep. If there's an imbalance in one of the rings in the circle below, your sleep can go off-kilter. We'll look at a different step in each chapter. Especially in the first three steps, knowing your Sleep Type – which we'll discuss as we move through this chapter – helps you to tailor your approach to repairing your sleep.

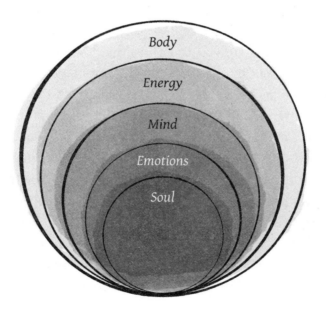

The Sleep Recovery Map is your guide to the programme: it works from the outside in and from the inside out. By that, I mean it works through the most physical to the most subtle aspects of your life to help you find the root of the problem. This way, you can take action to repair and heal the imbalances that sabotage your sleep.

Sleep Recovery principles, practices and people

As you go through the programme, you'll gather useful principles and powerful practices. You'll also hear about people whose stories might resonate with you. It makes sense that if you can't pinpoint what's sabotaging your sleep, you can't possibly know what to change to make it better. If you need to take on new practices, I'll explain why you need them, and how they work, with the best evidence available, giving you essential facts in a digestible way that respects your intelligence.

It's also true that what you practise – what you keep doing, day to day – is what you *become*. I'll give you specific, effective actions to take to repair your sleep – tools that create immediate and lasting change, to move you from sleeplessness to waking up happy. If you *do* the things that help you to be healthier and happier, you will bring yourself back into balance, reconditioning your body, brain, nervous system and reactions to life, so you can rest better at night and enjoy better days. I've spent years doing practices that support better health and I will tell you: they absolutely work. Once you learn how to move, breathe, manage your mind and emotions and connect inwardly, you'll wonder how you lived life without these tools.

As you get to know the people I describe in this book, look for the similarities between you and how you identify with all or part of their stories. This will help you find the tools and approaches most useful for you. Rather than calling people either 'owls' or 'larks', depending on whether they stay up late or wake early, I have found that there are three profiles that encompass the main sleep problems and their solutions. These are based on Ayurveda, a traditional Indian form of medicine born of close observation of people, which focuses not on simply treating symptoms but on creating underlying wellness. You'll see what worked for people who have a profile similar to your own. Though these are real-life examples, I have changed major details of each person's identity and joined stories together to create a composite picture to respect confidentiality.

Track your sleep

To identify your Sleep Type, you begin by tracking your sleep. If you went to a dietician, nutritionist or naturopath with a digestive problem, you'd be asked to track what you're eating, and the same principle applies to a sleep problem – sleep clinics and insomnia treatments start with checking the reality of your sleep situation. The Sleep Tracker I've created for you (see pages 24-25) draws upon the more traditional sleep diaries, and takes into account your daily habits, which can affect how well you get to sleep and stay asleep, and your energy throughout the day. There's a row to input the Sleep Recovery practices you'll integrate as you move through the steps of the programme: put a zero there to start, and when you start doing some practices, you'll start filling that bit in.

This is *not* meant to make you neurotic about your sleep habits, but to help you see where you can make progress relatively quickly by replacing sleep-sabotaging habits with sleep-supporting ones. You won't need to track your sleep forever – I'd suggest a month if you travel for work or have an irregular weekly pattern, but most people get a clear picture after two weeks.

Instead of tracking your sleep using an app or a device, I suggest you do it the old-fashioned way, using pen and paper. This keeps you off your phone or computer and encourages you to tune in to your internal rhythms and engage in the slower, physical act of recording them in writing. The sleep trackers you wear on your wrist in bed can only sense movement – they don't pick up your brainwaves or eye movements, which are needed to tell what phase of sleep you're in: it's not always true that deep sleep means no movement. Your heart rate may go up and you might move around a bit in the midst of deep, active dream-sleep; the tracker might label you as 'awake' when you're actually in a kind of very deep sleep, needed for restoring your mental well-being. Many people get very distressed about their sleep because of the inaccuracies of these tools, and that stress can make their sleep even worse!

Tracking your sleep by hand, based on your observations and an appraisal of how you feel, trains your senses, re-establishing a connection between your body, its needs and your behavioural patterns – rather than outsourcing your sense of self to a device. Keep the pages by your bed, or make a copy and keep it in your wallet if you are travelling.

Your sleep personality type

Particularly in the first three Sleep Recovery steps, you can identify and focus on the most valuable practices for you, using examples and a quiz to see which type describes you best.

I'm always surprised and intrigued at the many different ways people perceive and respond to conditions and situations in their lives: I hear from a diverse group of people as yoga therapist and psychotherapist. In the same situation, one person might get angry, while another will become despondent. What energises you might exhaust someone else. You may be thirsty for adventure, or you might feel happier with consistency. So while we are all unique and different, it's really useful to be aware of how basic constitutional and personality types can help us understand our sleep tendencies.

You have a basic constitution that stays with you throughout your life. Of course, you will change as you go through different life stages – adolescence, childbirth, menopause, ageing. Health conditions might crop up, but while these all play a role in shaping your body and how your personality is expressed, your constitution will make certain types of sleep imbalances more likely. In working with so many people's sleep problems, I've found the classification used in Ayurveda to be very helpful in explaining broad categories of physical, personality and sleep tendencies.

SLEEP MONKEY, TIGER OR BEAR?

Ayurveda classes people into predominant 'types' that relate human qualities of body and mind to the elements found in nature – namely fire, air, water and earth. While each person's combination of elements is unique, this way of looking at things clusters us into three main types. For the purposes of Sleep Recovery, I've associated an animal with each of these types because it may feel easier to relate to these than to the nature elements of Ayurveda. The Monkey type corresponds to the constitution that has airy qualities (in Ayurveda, called Vata), the Tiger type relates to a fiery constitution (Pitta), and the Bear represents the earthy-watery type (Kapha).

Monkey sleep problems: flitty, fractured and light sleep, anxious in nature, startled or unsettled. Vibrant, expansive mind, often light, weak or wiry body. 'Airy'

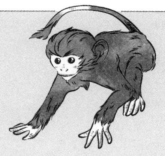

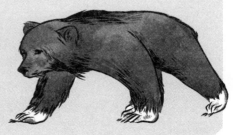

Tiger sleep problems: heavy sleep but far too little of it. Waking up too early or after just a few hours. Driven, overactive mind and/or body. 'Fiery'

Bear sleep problems: too much sleep, feeling sluggish and maybe sleeping too long with non-refreshing sleep. Can be depressive in nature, body can be slower moving. 'Earthy'

The Sleep Tracker	Monday	Tuesday	Wednesday
Sleep facts			
Wake time (today)			
Bed time (last night)			
Estimated time asleep			
Wakings in night			
Total hours asleep			
Habits and experience			
Dose and timing Caffeine Alcohol Nicotine Other stimulants (*see page* 80)			
Amount, type, timing Exercise Rest			
Sleep Recovery practices Morning wake-up Afternoon rest Pre-bedtime calming			
Daytime sleepiness			
Mood			
Additional factors: menstrual cycle, illness etc.			

Thursday	Friday	Saturday	Sunday

THE SLEEP TYPE QUIZ

The quiz below will help you to find your basic sleep tendencies and your Sleep Type so that you can focus on the most valuable actions you can take to repair your sleep at each step. Read each question, choose the answer that you identify with most and put a 1, 2 or 3 in the right-hand column. After answering all the questions, total up the number of 1s, 2s and 3s and you'll see which type you most identify with. Usually one number predominates: focus on that 'Sleep Type' as you go through the programme. If you relate to more than one type, just read the guidance for both – you can test which suggestions are more effective for you.

	Question	MONKEY 1	TIGER 2	BEAR 3	Number of your answer
sleep	What is your natural sleep tendency?	Light sleeper, tendency to wake in the night.	Little but sound, feel well rested with less than 8 hours.	Deep, prolonged, tend to wake up slowly.	
sleep problems	When your sleep is disturbed, what seems to be the main problem?	Can't get to sleep, very light sleep, feel I never get to sleep at all.	Can't stop activity at night, sleep a short time but not enough, wake too early, wake in the middle of the night, feel too activated to get back to sleep.	Can't seem to feel rested even after long sleep. Snoring/sleep apnoea/breathing problems.	
sleep characteristics	For this section, choose the statement that best describes your sleep.	I toss and turn in bed and feel restless. I can feel as though I've had no sleep all night.	I can have boundless energy in the middle of the night and find it hard to drop off to sleep.	Normally my sleep is heavy and prolonged. Sometimes I sleep too much and can wake up feeling groggy.	

	Question	MONKEY 1	TIGER 2	BEAR 3	Number of your answer
sleep characteristics	*For each section, choose the statement that best describes your sleep.*	It's hard for me to get to sleep, and when I do it's often interrupted. When I don't get enough sleep, I can feel dizzy and drowsy.	I get a burst of energy late at night, and like to read, watch movies or TV or do work.	I can often fall asleep right away during good times.	
		My insomnia is often tinged with anxiety and fear.	I find it hard to sleep unless I read a bit and then, when my eyes get tired, I can fall asleep with a book on my chest. I like to be busy with something right up until I fall asleep.	I can sleep most anywhere, and I love to sleep.	
		I find it difficult to get to sleep because my mind is buzzing.	I find it difficult to put down what I'm doing and go to bed.	I don't find it easy waking up after 8 hours.	
		I find it difficult to sleep in total darkness. I have a very active imagination, and darkness can make me anxious. I startle easily.	I don't like to sleep with any lights on. Light bothers my eyes. My sleep can be disturbed by small noises, even the sound of a watch ticking.	I can lack the energy to make it through the day.	

	Question	MONKEY 1	TIGER 2	BEAR 3	Number of your answer
sleep characteristics	For each section, choose the statement that best describes your sleep.	My sleep is variable and light, and I feel like I wake up several times in the night.	I tend to sleep less than the average 8 hours, but once I'm asleep my sleep can be very sound. I don't wake up loads in the night but often have a big wake-up: I may or may not be able to get back to sleep after this.	I can sleep long hours and still not feel rested, wanting naps and rests throughout the day.	
		I tend to be cold in my sleep.	I can feel like I'm overheating in my sleep or wake up sweating.	I am usually warm as I sleep.	
dreams	What are your dreams like, for the most part?	Quick, active, many, fearful.	Fiery, war, conflict/ violence.	Calm, romantic.	
body	How would you describe your general body type?	Slim, long limbs, angular, slight.	Medium, muscular.	Large – curvy or larger-set body.	
	How does your body deal with weight, for the most part?	Loses weight easily, more difficult to gain weight.	Gains and loses weight easily.	Gains easily, doesn't lose easily.	
	What is your general skin type?	Thin, dry, cold, rough.	Smooth, oily, warm, rosy.	Thick, oily, cool, pale.	
	What is the texture of your fingernails?	Dry, rough, brittle, break easily.	Sharp, flexible, pink, lustrous.	Thick, oily, smooth, shiny.	

	Question	MONKEY 1	TIGER 2	BEAR 3	Number of your answer
body	I'd describe my appetite, generally as:	Irregular, it comes and goes, I can forget to eat.	Generally good appetite, irritable when hungry.	Slow to mount appetite but steady.	
	My digestion is:	Irregular, I tend towards bloating/wind/ gassiness.	I digest quickly and can tend towards heartburn.	Digestion takes a while, and can be sluggish.	
	My thirst is:	Variable.	Always thirsty.	Not often thirsty.	
	My elimination is more like this:	Tends towards constipation.	Loose bowels.	Thick, sluggish bowel movement.	
energy	My physical energy can be described as, for my age group:	Hyperactive – always in motion.	Moderate – mobilises quickly in bursts of energy.	Slow – takes more to motivate and energy is steady once activated.	
	When I speak, I:	Speak quickly, can jump around, variable tone.	Speak pointedly, and in a penetrating way.	Use calm tones, can be slow and either not vary much in tone, or speak melodiously.	
mind	Mental energy	Hyperactive – I can be creative and move from one idea to another easily; I can have many projects on the go at one time and struggle to focus.	I can focus with intense attention and am quick to initiate projects but can run out of steam or become bored/not like finishing.	I can be slow to start projects but am patient, good at long-term problem-solving and completing projects.	

	Question	MONKEY 1	TIGER 2	BEAR 3	Number of your answer
mind	Memory	Good short-term memory.	Clear distinct memories.	Slow, sustained recollection.	
emotions	When I'm stressed:	I become anxious, fearful and uncertain.	I can get angry, irritable or aggressive.	I can become withdrawn, reclusive or stubborn.	
personality	I feel my personality is more:	Enthusiastic and energetic, clear-minded, quick-witted and supportive.	Generous, cheerful, humanitarian, success or leadership-oriented.	Joyful, warm, calm, peaceful and easy-going. I am a loving and steadying person to be around.	
	My worst traits are:	I can be 'spaced-out', flighty, indecisive, unaware or unfocused. I may have my head in the clouds, be 'hard to pin down' and forget or cancel plans.	I can be irritable, easily frustrated or impatient; can get angry, aggressive, overly focused on goals, controlling, manipulative, arrogant or self-centred.	I can be lazy, depressed, stuck and hard to motivate, overly attached/clingy, stubborn or closed-minded, and can refuse to 'let go'.	
	In work or relationships:	I enjoy change and variability.	I like to persuade or convince.	I like to support and to have consistency.	

	MONKEY	TIGER	BEAR
Total numbers for each type			

By now, you'll have a sense of your predominant Sleep Type. In the stories below, look for the experiences you can identify with, and you'll see how they relate to the problems for your Sleep Type and some possible solutions. You'll get a sense of how the Sleep Recovery programme worked for each person, and a preview of the tools you'll learn along the way that can help you. As you move through the steps, you'll hear more about Ollie, Liz and Cathy, as well as about some students and clients, and my own experiences.

Monkey Sleep Type: a live wire, airy

If you have difficulty falling asleep, staying asleep, or wake many times during the night, you may consider yourself to have a light, airy sleep type. People with an air-type constitution, even when they are in balance, tend to have lighter sleep. Personality-wise, air types can be creative or intellectual, in their heads, and often out of their bodies. Anxiety can be a symptom of being 'ungrounded' (see box), and when a person has suffered trauma their nervous system can respond by exhibiting these tendencies – it can feel fractured and disorganised. Air types tend to have long, lean limbs, and even if not thin can be bony or angular. They tend to have sparse appetites and can forget to eat, eat more lightly than average, and may be drawn towards raw or cold foods.

Practices that are focused on pulling energy or circulation downwards in the body, out of the head and bringing more awareness into the pelvis, legs and feet, are helpful. If you are an air type you may resist warming practices, heartier or warming foods and settling routines, but they are very healthy and balancing for this constitution.

Grounding

In yoga, grounding promotes *being* rather than *doing*. Grounding poses promote awareness of our physical and emotional connection with the Earth and bring a feeling of calm and balance, especially useful for 'scattered' people who live in their heads.

OLLIE: A MONKEY TYPE

Ollie had a tall frame and high cheekbones. His slightly rounded shoulders, pale skin and hollow eye sockets gave him a slightly vampiric look. Ollie was a single man in his mid-40s, who came to me when he was regularly getting less than three hours of sleep a night. He could push through his day but often disconnected from his work colleagues. After he missed a series of meetings (they just slipped his mind) and then snapped at a colleague, the HR director at work passed him my business card – she'd been to one of my 'yoga for insomnia' workshops and thought Ollie might get some relief. As a software engineer, he had an active intellect, and dealt well with abstract ideas. He would often work into the night without eating a meal, consumed with a coding problem at work. He'd been consulting at the company for almost a year but when offered a permanent contract he'd turned it down – he didn't like feeling pinned down.

Ollie spent what free time he had devouring novels or running near-marathon distances several times per week – mostly in the early hours of the morning or late at night, after a dinner of salad at his desk. The sleeping tablet prescribed by his doctor wasn't really working any more. He would run long distances to try to tire himself out, but often fell asleep at 2 a.m. for about 90 minutes followed by very light sleep, as though he were hovering above his sheets.

In our first week, Ollie started the sleep tracker and I taught

Tiger Sleep Type: fiery in nature

If you have a fiery nature, it can be hard to get to sleep because you're doing too much. You can wake with a start early in the morning with high levels of stress hormones in your system, needing little to jolt you out of bed. Fiery types tend towards shorter, deeper bursts of sleep.

Fiery types can have strong personalities, gravitate towards leadership and be highly motivated. They can quickly display anger, him the Simple Sleep Sequence (see page 42). I watched as his body seemed to drop into the yoga poses more deeply – it was as though he'd become heavier. His breath was freer and longer and his face and eyes softened.

Over the weeks we worked together, Ollie began to eat more warming foods, making a large soup or stew at home to eat in the office in the evenings. He began to leave work a bit earlier, planned to eat earlier in the evening, and created a winding-down routine at the end of the day, which involved leaving his phone outside his bedroom and reading a book before doing the Simple Sleep Sequence and going to bed. He began to exercise during the day, taking a lunch hour to do so. He stopped having caffeine in the afternoon, instead doing a brief meditation or the Feet Up and Rest position in his office chair (you'll learn about these in Steps 1 and 2.) Ollie initially lived alone, keeping unsociable hours. I bumped into him a year and a half after his last session with me. He had gained some weight, which suited him, had taken a full-time position at his company, and although he said he still slept lightly, he slept more regular hours, drank a lot less coffee, and no longer needed sleeping pills. He was proud to tell me that he'd found out, to his delight, that he doesn't snore, according to his girlfriend of over a year. The routines and 'grounding' helped him to keep doing the things he loved, to balance them out and add some more nourishment to his life.

impatience, resentment or frustration. People with this constitution can seem to have boundless energy and may need to expend some of this energy – to *discharge* it – before they can properly relax. They may also desperately need to balance the exhaustion that can come from 'firing on all cylinders'. Fiery types tend to be more muscular and can gain or lose weight relatively quickly when their bodies are in good balance. They tend to have a strong appetite, a directional walk and an intense gaze.

LIZ: A TIGER TYPE

Liz, 56, a professor at a business school, was heavily involved in local politics and a married mother of two. She was funny, sharp and spoke in rapid-fire sentences, with intensity and humour. She was a natural leader, fuelled by a powerful history of family hardship. Her face held tension as she sat forwards in her seat, armed with a small red notebook from which she reported back her 'bad nights' with barely a pause for breath between sentences.

At the start of the six-week course she attended with me, Liz was sleeping poorly six nights each week, struggling to fall asleep, often waking with a start in the middle of the night and not getting back to sleep. On the seventh night she rested reasonably well, but not enough to make up for the previous six. After 25 years of success at work and in local politics, she began having panic attacks about both. She'd then met a friend from university for a drink and, hearing her story, Liz's friend had insisted that she attend one of my courses. Though Liz was definitely not a 'yoga person', she was desperate enough to try it.

After the first week's session, Liz reported back with surprise that doing the Simple Sleep Sequence (see page 42) nightly was easy and it had really helped her relax before bed. She'd slept through the night more easily. Over the six weeks, I helped her to focus on breathing less forcefully and more smoothly. We reviewed the stretches I'd given her to do, and chose some from the sequence that would be most helpful if she did happen to wake in the middle of the night. Her sleep improved dramatically and the breathing and stretches helped her to slow down – and cool down – before sleep, as well as feel calmer in the daytime.

Liz reported a 70 per cent improvement in her sleep after the group course, but wanted to 'knock the problem on the head' and asked questions specifically related to menopause in one-to-one sessions. We began by reviewing her physical habits, then her nervous system patterning and how she managed stress, and we talked about life transition issues. One particular point stays with me: 'Do I really have to give up wine and coffee?' she asked. My reply: 'If it's causing sleep problems, and if you want to sleep better, let it go, even if just for now.' Quitting coffee in favour of a single cup of tea before 11 a.m. made a massive difference. Her sleep tracking also showed that middle-of-the-night wake-ups were likelier if she had even a single glass of wine in the evening. Learning how caffeine, alcohol and other habits would affect her sleep made a big difference for Liz: she needed a credible, rational explanation for why she should change her habits. You'll find this information in Step 1 (see page 82).

Liz kept up the yoga poses each night, feeling deeply relaxed after her 10-minute practice. I helped make sure she was breathing slowly enough, as her natural tendency was always to speed up! Breathing more slowly helped lower her stress during the day as well. You'll learn about this in Step 2 (see page 92).

Liz saw the benefits of the Simple Sleep Sequence and continued to make simple and useful changes in her sleep and in her life, following each step in the programme. Given her active, fiery mind, Step 3 – focused on the mind – was particularly powerful for her. When she added Sleep Recovery meditation practices to her day, her energy became more stable; her sleep was deeper and more reliable.

As she integrated the practices at every step of the programme, I noticed she'd enter the room more and more calmly, and when I see her occasionally now, she sits back with ease, and her brow is no longer furrowed. She insisted her Sleep Recovery had been 'better than Botox' for her appearance. She still laughed easily – and more heartily than ever. We'll see Liz again in discussions about wine, and meditation.

Addressing the over-exertion of the fire type is essential, so practices that slow down and rebalance the tendency towards the fight or flight/stress response can be especially beneficial. Habits, practices and foods that are 'cooling and soothing' tend to work well to balance this type of person.

Balancing

In yoga, balancing is about *smoothing* out the bursts of adrenaline that a fiery person can experience, and harnessing a sense of sustainable energy. This is a physical and emotional connection with the soothing qualities of water and the grounding qualities of earth, especially useful for helping the highly motivated to learn to recharge and rest.

Bear Sleep Type: a slow and steady, earthy/watery type

If you have an earthier or more watery constitution, you're more likely to sleep deeply and/or for a long time. However, when these types of people are out of balance, they can sleep or rest for a long time but feel unrefreshed, groggy or sluggish.

This type tends to be generous and home-oriented with relatively more stability in life, but can tend towards stubbornness or feeling stuck. Those with a more earthy constitution may be more 'grounded' but can tip into inertia or laziness. The slowest-moving of the constitution types, people in this category tend to metabolise food more slowly so they can keep weight more easily. They tend towards a more rounded, full or curvy physique, thick hair and, when in balance, shining eyes.

It's essential to get enough exercise and activation to allow for deep and effective sleep. For those who tend to be more earthy, it's important to do sweat-inducing cardio activity in the morning or afternoon to build up the appetite for sleep. Relatively less emphasis on *grounding* and more on *elevating* practices during the day are helpful.

CATHY: A BEAR TYPE

Cathy was retired, and had practised gentle yoga at home for most of her adult life as her main form of exercise. She enjoyed yoga because by moving her body she found some relief from a general low mood that could tip into a depressive state in autumn and winter, especially after her husband died. She would feel lethargic and sluggish, and sometimes during the dark months she'd not get to sleep until 2 or 3 a.m. She'd try to catch up on sleep, staying in bed late, but rarely felt rested. She felt little spark and struggled with low energy.

Cathy loved participating in a group class – meeting people of all ages and knowing she wasn't alone in her insomnia helped her feel less isolated, and she found that connecting with other people helped dissolve both her loneliness and her sleep anxiety. She used the Sleep Tracker (see pages 24–25) and fed back on her progress each week, asking questions and getting support and suggestions for refinement.

Cathy did the Simple Sleep Sequence (see page 42) every night, which helped her to feel ready to sleep. Doing bedtime yoga not only helped her to get to sleep, but also helped her to sleep more deeply and soundly, waking more refreshed in the morning. If she became drowsy and went to bed skipping the pre-sleep stretches, she was more apt to wake in the middle of the night or to sleep more fitfully.

I encouraged Cathy to move her body more vigorously than she normally did in her home yoga practice during the day. She did some energising wake-up breathing and moves (see Step 2) that she learned: these were a real revelation for her, especially the Breath of Joy (see page 103). Her new morning routine gave her a lot more spark throughout the day. To her delight, Cathy's children noticed she had more energy as she played with her grandchildren and after a few months of better sleep, she began volunteering with a local charity, which helped her feel more purposeful and less lonely. We will hear more about Cathy later.

Elevating

In yoga, elevating or energising is about *activating* the body and mind, especially during the daytime. Elevating poses are empowering: mobilising our physical and emotional connection with the internal, transformative fire; bringing a feeling of purpose, especially useful for sluggish people who tend towards low mood.

While you may not fit all the characteristics for one just one sleep profile or relate to *all* the traits listed for the type you most identify with, using the three types can help you focus your Sleep Recovery on your specific needs, particularly in the first three steps. And now let's get to work on your sleep transformation!

STEP 1

Repair your body

AS WE AGREED in the previous chapter, you're not a machine, and going to sleep isn't like switching from 'on' to 'off'. You move from an intentional state, in which you're actively doing things, into a state in which the natural, automatic processes in your body take over. This step shows you how.

When all goes well, your body knows *exactly* what to do. A symphony of hormones plays through you, aligned to daylight and darkness cues, helping you to feel drowsy when it's time to sleep, orchestrating a series of movements throughout your waking and sleeping life. Your brainwave patterns, heart rate and breath change over the course of a night's sleep, a series of variations on a theme. The tune changes when the wake-up call sounds. When things are working, these rhythms and melodies happen of their own accord, and nature takes its course.

This step helps you to be *in tune* with your body by removing the armour of muscle tension and bringing back the naturally relaxed body that glides into a good night's sleep. I'm excited for you, because once you learn these tools and how to use them, you'll see how you much power you have to change how you feel – and like all the tools in this programme, once you learn them they are yours to use forever: anywhere, any time, whenever you need them they'll be there. This step has two parts:

Part 1: You'll learn the **Basic Yoga Breath**, which you'll use during your sleep prep and to balance your nervous system throughout the day (we'll cover this in more detail in Step 2). This breath works in partnership with the **Simple Sleep Sequence**, a set of movements that dissolve the *tension* in your body that's built up throughout the day. It prepares you for sleep, or helps you back to sleep if you wake in the middle of the night (see page 41). Your body will have its particular way of holding tension. While the sequence covers your whole body, once you learn it you can see which postures are the most beneficial to you and zero in on those areas if you're shorter on time.

Part 2: You'll learn about how sleep works, the most common sleep saboteurs, and how to stop doing the things that you may not have realised were actively undermining your sleep. I'll show you how your habits throughout the day affect your sleep at night so that you can stop doing the things that damage your sleep, while not getting obsessive or fixated on your habits – you'll slowly put in the good things and the harmful things will fall away more easily. You'll get your day back in sync with how your body evolved to work, and incorporate some good, simple habits. This is often called 'sleep hygiene' but I think it's just part of generally living well. Instead of just telling you what to do, I think it's important that you know how caffeine, alcohol, electronic screens and other habits affect your sleep so that you can make good decisions and take action.

PART 1:
THE SIMPLE SLEEP SEQUENCE: RELEASE TENSION AND SETTLE YOUR BODY

If I've been sitting down to work for a while, it's not until I stand up that I realise how tight my shoulders have become and how stagnant my whole body feels. When I stretch my arms out and start moving around I feel broader, brighter and more present. We often discount the tension that builds up in our bodies throughout the day, and how important it is to peel it off like you might shed your work clothes at the end of the day, or change from outdoor clothes into something softer and more comfortable.

The Simple Sleep Sequence helps you find the places you're holding tension and melt them down: you will soften and expand your breathing, which will directly affect your mind and how you feel. Think back to the Sleep Recovery Map on page 19: the outside rings affect the inside rings, and vice versa. You'll be better able to feel *and respond to* the changes in your energy throughout the day, and get yourself in line with the day's natural rhythm.

Here's how it works: your mind has a great deal of say in how your body feels, but it's a two-way relationship. Your body sends strong messages to your brain, guiding it in how to react on a primal level, creating a neurochemical environment in your brain that affects your mood and influences your sleep. Your body is designed to tighten against threat – to protect you. The problem is that this tensed-up and protective state can easily become chronic, and long after highly stressful events have passed, your body can carry a lot of unnecessary tension, affecting not only your musculature but also your body's hormonal functioning. In other words, tension sabotages your sleep by 'breaking' the mechanisms of relaxation. The same body-to-brain signalling can also be used to communicate that it's okay to relax. So the good news is that you can change your *body* to change your mind, setting off a chain reaction of positive sleep-readying behaviour.

Another key to Sleep Recovery is restoring your ability to feel the tiredness cues that happen naturally when you're in sync with nature – allowing yourself to feel tired, and acknowledging that tiredness. This is part of a capacity called 'interoception', which is our internal sense of ourselves – our long-evolved responses to the innate needs for safety, food, water and rest. When interoception is broken, we lose our ability to sense and respond to danger, overwhelm, thirst, hunger and tiredness. Our daily lives may force us to do this to ourselves bit by bit every day, or we may have experienced a trauma or been subject to conditions that mean we have lost this sense (discussed in more detail in Step 4), so our need to sleep and rest is broken as well. When you are taut with tension, your body naturally *feels* less – it's stuck in the fight or flight response.

This step helps you to bring back sensation and body awareness, so that you can better respond to your body's cues throughout the day. When you pull the tension out of your muscles, you will experience a calmer, more responsive body, which signals to your brain that you are more relaxed. Let's now learn about soothing, softening, releasing and relaxing to restore sensation and finer awareness of your internal state.

The Simple Sleep Sequence

Use this sequence of movements to repair the relationship between your body, breath and brain, learning to listen to your body's needs. All of the sleep preparation practices reduce physical tension, lower your heart rate, and decrease the stress hormones in your body. Doing them in your bedroom can make the room a calm and soothing space as you prepare for sleep.

Simple Sleep Sequence: The exercises

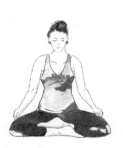
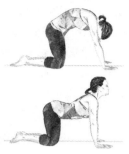
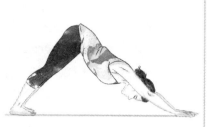

1 Basic Yoga Breath   **2** Cat / Cow Pose   **3** Downward Dog

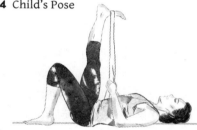
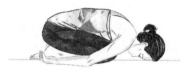
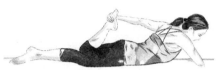

4 Child's Pose   **5** Quad Stretch

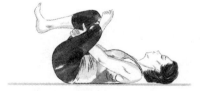
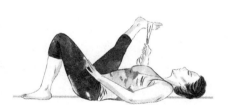

6 Hamstring Stretch   **7** Extended Inner Thigh Stretch

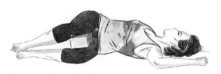

8 Outer Hip Stretch   **9** Simple Spinal Twist

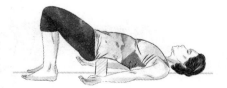
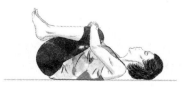

10 Supported Little Bridge Pose   **11** Knees to Chest Pose

This series of movements, especially when combined with the Basic Yoga Breath, below, or the lengthened-exhale settling breath (in Step 2), helps to relax the essential areas of your body needed to get to sleep. This series of movements takes about 20–25 minutes when you're first learning it and about 10–12 minutes when it's become routine, even if you're doing it slowly. It doesn't become less effective with continued use, as sleeping pills do. Instead, the more you practise it, the better you'll become at getting a deeper and more releasing stretch.

Before you start, grab a yoga brick (a couple of thick, heavy books will do just as well) and a yoga belt (or a strong sash from a bathrobe or a long belt). Just make sure the belt you use isn't stretchy. It needs to be firm so that you can press out against it.

1 Basic Yoga Breath

* Breathe in and out through your nose only (with your mouth closed).
* Intentionally create the sound you'd make when yawning or sighing by gently contracting/tightening the back of your throat to make a hissing sound (you'll find more on how to do this when we learn about ujjayii breath on page 92). This lets less air through and streamlines the flow of your breath.
* This tone in your throat, combined with lengthening your exhale, activates the 'rest and digest' part of your nervous system (parasympathetic), creating more relaxation in your body and mind. You'll learn more about this in Step 2.

2 Cat Pose and Cow Pose

◆ Come up on all fours into a box position and spread your fingers out to open your hands.

◆ Keep your wrists under your shoulders (or just in front of them if your wrists feel tight) and your knees under your hips.

◆ Take a slow, deep breath in, arching your back and opening the front of your chest. This is cow pose.

◆ With a long steady exhale, draw your belly in and down, rounding the back and stretching between your shoulder blades. This is cat pose.

◆ Keep your eyes and forehead relaxed as you do this – you can even close your eyes if you prefer.

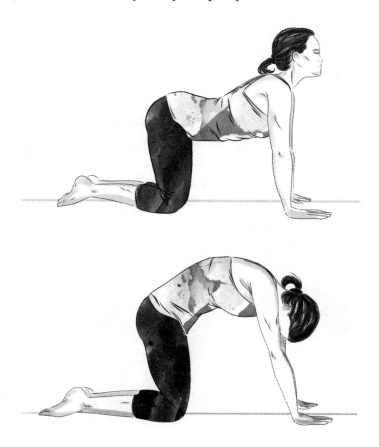

STEP 1: REPAIR YOUR BODY

This pose stretches the muscles between your ribs, making space for you to breathe. It is also said to tone the vagus nerve, which runs from the back of your skull down into your torso, passing through all the major internal organs. It's responsible for body-to-brain messaging between your heart and other internal organs, which signals whether your body is relaxed or agitated. This set of slow movements sends the relaxation message.

Slow breathing and rhythmic movement done together calm and soothe your nervous system. Keep the Basic Yoga Breath throughout the sequence, and when you find you've forgotten to breathe like this, just start again.

BACK LENGTHENERS AND THIGH STRETCH

From an all-fours position, hands and knees on your mat or on the floor, you can do either or both of these poses.

3 Downward Dog

◆ For a more intense full-body stretch, move from all fours into the position called Downward Dog, the inverted V shape, by lifting your knees off the floor and walking your feet back behind your pelvis.

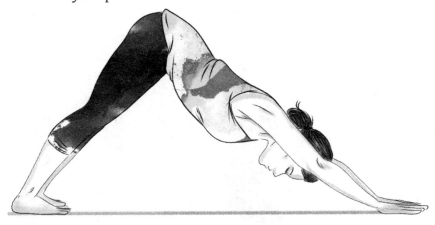

- Press your hips upwards and back so that your bottom forms the angle of the inverted V, pressing your chest back towards your legs.
- Keep your arms straight and fingers spread evenly.
- Relax your neck: keep the back of your neck long.

This pose re-establishes good circulation and stretches in the longest body muscles: hamstrings, shoulders, spinal support muscles and neck. Placing your head below your heart calms your mind, and being inverted (upside down) brings circulation to your chest – and with plenty of oxygen, your body feels more balanced and refreshed.

4 Child's Pose

- From a box position, bring your big toes together and widen your knees apart.
- Bring your bottom down towards your heels. If this is too much strain on your hips, roll up a blanket and place it beneath your bottom. Let your arms rest by your sides.
- With your forehead on the floor, press the flesh of your forehead downward towards your nose – this releases the frontalis muscle in your forehead, which feeds back a *calm* signal to your nervous system.
- Breathe here: visualise your breath moving up the back of your body as you inhale, and down the front as you exhale. Stay here for 5 to 10 breaths, or longer if you wish.

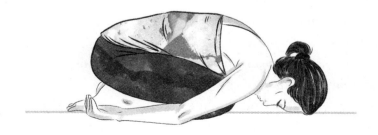

This pose can be used on its own or after Downward Dog/inverted V shape, after which you slowly lower your knees to the floor. This pose lengthens your back muscles and the back of your pelvis, and can feel very calming and soothing. It's a pose that many young children discover on their own as a way to re-centre when they feel overwhelmed.

Cathy particularly loved the opening Cat and Cow stretches and the Downward Dog pose, which helped her feel her breath come to life and move her circulation around her body more easily. Downward Dog powered up her arms and legs.

Liz found that Downward Dog helped to tire out her arms and legs, and after holding the pose as long as she could, she felt more relaxed.

Ollie loved being in Child's Pose, and gently rocked his forehead back and forth on the floor, smoothing his brow: it felt to him like clearing his thoughts and calming his brain.

5 Quad Stretch

- Lie face-down with the tops of your feet pressing into the floor.
- Lift your chest and place your right forearm on the floor in front of you for support.
- Bend your left knee and grab the top of your left foot with your left hand. If you can't reach your foot, use a scarf or belt looped around your left foot.
- Keep the left side of your torso long by breathing deeply and extending your body.
- Keep squeezing your thighs towards the midline of your body and keep your glutes engaged without gripping.

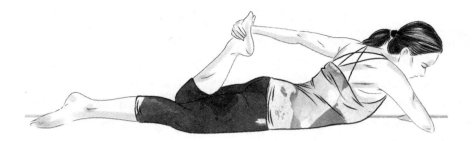

- Pull your lower belly away from the floor to engage your abdominal muscles – this will support your back so it doesn't feel compressed or painful.
- Direct your bottom down towards your heels – this will deepen the stretch and support your lower back.
- To intensify the stretch, press your left foot back into your left hand as you draw that foot towards your bottom.
- Pause for a moment between sides, feeling the difference between the stretched left leg and the right leg. This builds your capacity to sense changes in your body over time.
- Now switch sides and repeat with the right leg.

This move stretches the muscles that go from the front of your hip through the bulk of your thigh into the knee. Keeping your knee in line with your bottom keeps you from straining your knee.

Front-of-thigh stretches are vital – thighs are often forgotten and can be incredibly tight. You have four muscles here, hence the name 'quadriceps' (four-heads). The muscle group runs from your pelvis to just below your knee, and when tight it can pull your low back out of alignment, causing pain and creating tension in your pelvis and lower abdomen. By relaxing your quads, you bring circulation down into your lower body and create the releasing and broadening action needed to initiate relaxation.

LEG RELEASE SERIES

This series of three stretches releases your hamstrings (the bane of the runner's or cyclist's existence), opens up the often-tight inner thigh and releases the glutes and outer hip. Basically, it rebalances the circulation in your hips and pelvis and helps alleviate low back pain. It also helps relieve any fluid retention, swelling or stagnation in your legs. This opens up the muscles so that the nerve pathways into the lower abdominal organs, as well as the inner thigh and sacral (lower back) areas, can function better. Excellent for those who sit in chairs all day, drive or travel a lot. And finally, these stretches help you feel grounded and ready for sleep. You'll need a belt for poses 6 and 7.

6 Hamstring Stretch

◆ Lie on your back with your knees bent and the soles of your feet on the floor. Keep your lower back gently curved, so that the natural arch is present in the spine, leaving a little space between the lower back and the floor. You'll use this same 'neutral' position for all three poses in this series.

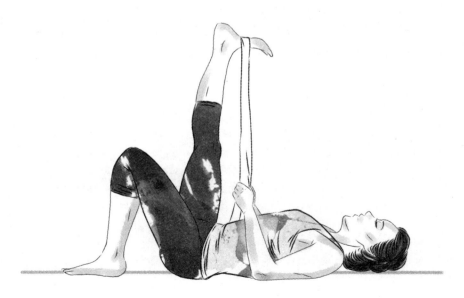

- Extend your right leg up towards the ceiling and push the ball of your foot into the belt, keeping the knee unlocked.
- Pull down on the belt with your hands, *keeping your elbows on the floor with your shoulders relaxed.*
- Press your thigh bone away from your chest so your leg straightens more, and keep breathing into your lower abdomen. Every exhalation will enable you to stretch a bit deeper – stretch enough to notice a difference but not so much that you cause yourself to tense up.
- When you feel a good stretch in the hamstring, move on to the next pose, staying on the same leg for the next two movements.

7 Extended Inner Thigh Stretch

- Move your right leg out to the side, towards the floor – don't try to get the extended leg all the way to the floor. If your pelvis tilts and your opposite hip raises, you'll miss the inner thigh stretch.
- Keep your arms relaxed and your elbows resting on the floor as you pull back on the belt with your hand to intensify the inner leg stretch. Breathe smoothly, with the exhale a little longer than the inhale. Move on to the third part when you've felt a release in the muscle.

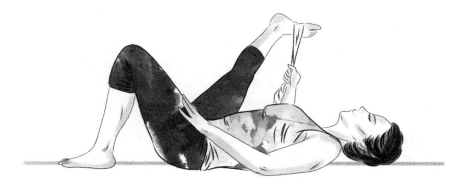

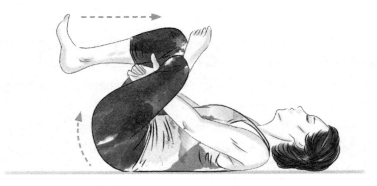

8 Outer Hip Stretch

♦ Flex your right foot to engage the calf muscle and support the knee. Bend your left knee and cross your right ankle over the top of the other thigh (NB: the image above shows your left ankle on top of the knee – it's easier to visualise this way, but as I mentioned on page 51, you should do the whole sequence on your right leg before switching legs).

♦ Wrap your top hip downwards, following the arrows in the picture, moving the sitting bone in your bottom down towards your tailbone.

♦ Draw in the lower knee towards your chest to intensify the stretch.

♦ Resist away with the rotated leg by moving your hip down, rather than pressing into your knee.

Hip stretches help to concentrate attention and circulation into your lower body, bringing blood flow into your lower digestive tract area. When the muscles around your digestive tract are tense and tight, this may decrease blood flow and cause constriction that affects the gut's ability to absorb nutrients and move our food along properly. We now know a great deal of the essential neurochemicals needed for mental health and balanced sleep originate here, in the gut.

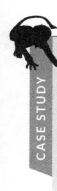
Ollie, the Monkey-type sleeper, who tended to feel ungrounded and 'in his head', particularly loved the leg stretches and hip openers while breathing deeply and rhythmically into his lower abdomen. As a runner, releasing his legs and hips made him feel much calmer and more settled.

Coming to your senses

After completing the Leg Release Series on one side, pause before changing legs to notice the difference in sensation between the side you've just stretched and the one that has not yet been stretched. This interoception (body awareness) pause can be very valuable in helping you come to recognise what your body feels like when it is properly relaxed versus how it feels normally. Many of my students report after doing the thigh, leg and hip stretches that they feel heavier or calmer, more expansive or warmer on the side they've stretched as compared with the un-stretched leg. The contrast tells you something about the difference between a calm body and a keyed-up body. This helps to develop the important sense of interoception – your conscious awareness of your body's state of tension, relaxation, safety, danger, hunger, sleepiness etc.

9 Simple Spinal Twist

◆ Roll completely to your left side and bend your knees, bringing them up in line with your hip bone, keeping your outer right hip and outer right knee resting on the floor.
◆ Stack your right leg evenly on top of the left, matching up your knees. Squeeze a yoga block or cushion between your knees to keep the joints in your lower back even.

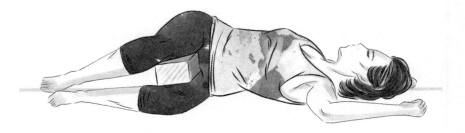

• Keeping your lower body stable in this position, twist from your middle and upper back, broadening your left shoulder to the left.

• Breathing smoothly and lengthening your exhale, let your upper back spread out and settle your right shoulder closer to the floor.

• Breathe with awareness of the middle rib cage area, expanding as you inhale and softening as you exhale. You'll learn about this more in Step 2 (see page 97).

• To come out of the pose, bring your knees up to your chest and hug them with your arms. Then roll on to the other side and do the pose there before moving on to the next posture.

Like many twisting yoga postures, this pose releases your shoulders, neck, upper back, and the long muscles that line your spine. It is particularly effective on the muscles along your thoracic spine, in the middle back, which relaxes the upper back/shoulders. This

Posture tip

Using a block or cushion between your knees for this pose is especially important if you have any lower back pain or have had an injury there. This means you're stabilising the joint so that the muscles above it can mobilise, lengthen and broaden, which helps alleviate back pain by taking the strain off the joint.

Liz, with her more fiery constitution, was particularly fond of the twisting poses. They helped to release the tension in her shoulders and free up her breath. She also noticed that her stomach settled more easily after opening up the 'solar plexus' area. The neck stretch alleviated the eyestrain and the tension headache she'd get from long hours at the computer.

pose also opens your chest, giving you more breathing space. Since most of us are in a hunched-forward position for much of the day – driving, picking up children, working at a computer, carrying heavy bags or crouching over a mobile phone – releasing the tension you carry here is key. This also frees up the muscles between your ribs, the intercostals. When these are tight, they inhibit your breathing and lock in the physiological tension response. When you open up this area, you will naturally breathe more easily and feel freer.

It works particularly well with the middle-ribcage breath explained as part of three-part breath (see page 98). This pose is one of my absolute favourites because it opens up the area around my stomach, where I hold a lot of tension from sitting down at a computer all day. If you have a lot of anxiety, you may find this area very tense, and this stretch can feel like a massive relief.

The pose is also great because it lengthens the hard-to-stretch muscles that run from your lower back to your shoulders. The twisting gently compresses and then releases the tissue around your digestive organs, which can feel like you're flushing the area, while releasing tension from your abdominal muscles.

10 Supported Little Bridge Pose

This pose, in which you lift your lower back just a couple of inches off the floor with some support (a thick book or a yoga block), is best done on the floor, or on a firm mattress.

* Lie on your back with your knees bent, soles of the feet to the floor and knees pointing up to the ceiling with a gentle curve in your lower back, as you did for the Leg Release Series (see page 50).
* Place your ankles directly under your knees, with your feet parallel.
* Keep your abdominal muscles, thighs and bottom gently engaged – but not tense – as you lift your hips up to halfway between your knees and your heart.
* Breathe into the centre of your chest, keep the sides of your torso long, and bring your shoulder blades towards one another on your back to expand your chest.
* Rest the sacrum area of your lower back (the triangular plate of bone at the base of your spine) on a yoga block on its lowest setting, which is about 7.5–10cm (3–4in) high – keep your hips substantially lower than your knees.

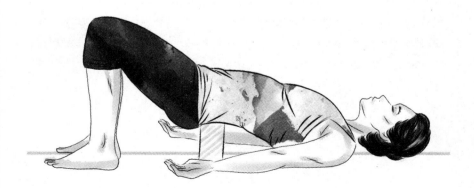

◆ Keep breathing into your ribcage while resting in this pose for 1–5 minutes. To come out of it, activate your leg muscles, pressing your feet into the floor, and lift your bottom away from the block. Then rest with your lower back on the floor for a few breaths before the last posture.

This is a gentle and not overly stimulating stretch for the chest (pectoral muscles), which gets very tight from stress or from a hunched-forward position. It opens up your diaphragm and lengthens the abdominal muscles. This position also increases circulation to your throat, where the thyroid and parathyroid reside. These two glands relate to the hormones that regulate digestion and sleep.

This pose also works by putting pressure on the 'baroreceptors' located at the top of the lungs, which may account for the way it seems to stimulate the 'relaxation response' so well and so quickly for many of my clients.

It opens up your breathing, which is really important because when you don't breathe well, you don't sleep well. Your body is evolutionarily adapted to remain alert if there is any inhibition or constraint in your breathing, because your body is very well aware that when you can't breathe, you can't stay alive.

It's one of my favourites – with my sacrum resting on a block, it creates just the right angle to lower my heart rate quickly and I find myself immediately 'dropping in' to a more relaxed state.

Posture tip

Keep the natural curve at the back of your neck – don't flatten your neck. Make sure you can breathe easily with no strain in your neck or face.

11 Knees to Chest Pose

◆ Lying on your back, draw your knees inward towards your chest and take several breaths to lengthen your lower back.

◆ If you're practising on the floor instead of a bed, some small slow circular rolls, gently pressing your lower back into the floor as you draw your knees in and arching as your knees move away from your chest, can feel very relaxing – like the rocking action that sends infants to sleep.

◆ Place your palms on your kneecaps and let your legs drop away from your torso as much as possible without losing your grip. This massages the tailbone area.

◆ Roll in small circles to release tension in the muscle-to-bone connections along the sacrum, which supports relaxation and grounding.

This pose creates a balance to the back-bending action of the previous front-body-opening pose. And you're on your back, so it's easy to settle into a sleeping position from here if you're doing this on your bed. I find it both soothing and containing. If you prefer it, you can substitute the first pose in the sequence, Child's Pose.

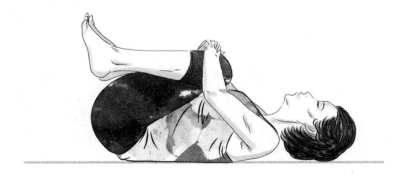

The Simple Sleep Sequence is a full-body comforting routine, once you get the hang of it. Depending on where you hold your tension, you may discover after doing the sequence several times that certain moves are your favourites: they do the trick for you, helping you to relax quickly and easily. I find that doing the ones my body needs most (often the quad stretch and the twist, other times the hamstring stretch and the gentle backbend) can be a quick way to relax my body, and I've come to sense what my body needs most. I also add new stretches if I have extra time. I don't see this as an obligation, but as a daily treat, unravelling my body before bed.

Creature comfort: shaking out the tension

Recently, I was in a crowded café, and noticed a Jack Russell terrier seated next to a woman having coffee. The dog's eyes darted from side to side and seemed to widen as the noise levels in the room rose – the bell on the door clanging, the espresso grinder going, a baby crying, and another dog barking. Little Jack was clearly well trained to rest patiently and behave, but was visibly overstimulated, as his eyes widened and tension seemed to mount. When his owner patted his head and neck, he shook himself out and then settled back to sit, looking visibly more relaxed.

Two things happened in that moment – comforting touch and unashamedly, un-self-consciously shaking out tension. These are key to regulating the stress levels in our own bodies. These are also things that humans, especially in our mostly stressful, highly regulated context – the workplace – have been socialised away from doing.

The Simple Sleep Sequence and many of the practices in this book give you ways to peel off tension when you feel it arise, and to actually become more conscious of where tension mounts in your body throughout the day. You may start to notice that you'll more spontaneously get up and move around as you need, adding in stretches throughout the day once you've got into the habit – as a form of self-soothing and connection to your body.

PART 2:
STOP SABOTAGING
YOUR SLEEP

The next part of bringing your body back into balance to recover your sleep involves noticing and shifting the habits that sabotage your sleep.

First, you need to understand and get back on track with the natural rhythms of the day and how your body responds to these. Then you'll learn what changes in work patterns, light and darkness, caffeine, alcohol and screen time may be doing to undermine your sleep so you can make sleep-supporting choices.

Human beings follow a roughly 24-hour cycle called the circadian rhythm (circa = around, diem = day – the cycles move *around the day),* which responds primarily to light and darkness cues with physical, mental and behavioural changes. If your natural rhythms are disrupted by going to bed at the wrong time, changing time zones, or high stress levels, you may be running counter to the way our sleep, as a species, evolved. If you're fighting millions of years of evolution, it's no wonder you are having trouble sleeping.

Many of us become sleepy not long after it's fully dark outside, but disregard the instinct to sleep. Maybe you keep your bedtime constant regardless of the season, and if you're like many people, this may be far later than the most beneficial bedtime for your body. I have noticed that I become tired well before what I consider an acceptable bedtime – a bit after sunset, when it's dark out, irrespective of the season. This is when we'd naturally start making our way to sleep. We most often override this and find ourselves getting a second wind, which prevents us from getting to sleep when we had intended to.

Your light-activated body clock

....

How does light affect our sleep? A bundle of about 20,000 nerve cells in your brain acts as a biological 'master clock', setting off reactions in response to daylight and darkness. If all works as it should, at the end of the day the fading light and growing darkness spark a sleep-inducing chain reaction throughout your whole body. Your eyes convey the message to the master clock, which, through a few steps, gets in touch with the pineal gland. This then nudges your brain to convert *serotonin* (one of the most well-known neurotransmitters, sometimes called 'the happy hormone') into *melatonin*, which readies you for sleep by making you drowsy, decreasing your core body temperature – an important (if counter-intuitive) factor in making you drowsy (see page 65). If you then look at bright light or heat your body up too much, you confuse the signals, and, for some people, the sleep-inducing chain reaction is thrown into chaos.

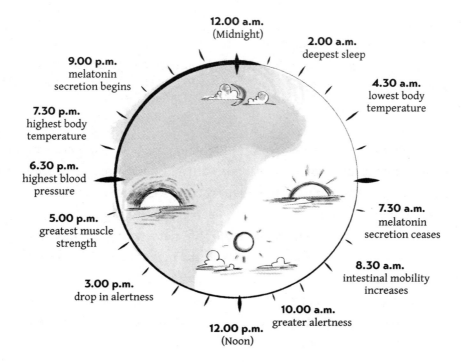

12.00 a.m.
(Midnight)

2.00 a.m.
deepest sleep

9.00 p.m.
melatonin
secretion begins

4.30 a.m.
lowest body
temperature

7.30 p.m.
highest body
temperature

6.30 p.m.
highest blood
pressure

7.30 a.m.
melatonin
secretion ceases

5.00 p.m.
greatest muscle
strength

8.30 a.m.
intestinal mobility
increases

3.00 p.m.
drop in alertness

10.00 a.m. greater alertness

12.00 p.m.
(Noon)

Another tendency is for our bodies to experience a slump in energy in the early afternoon. This occurs naturally as part of the circadian rhythm, with a temporary dip in core body temperature triggering a release of melatonin, and our level of response to it depends on how long we've been awake and whether we were already in a sleep-deprived state. Most of us learn to push past 'the 3 p.m. slump': if we're at work or running around doing errands when it hits, rather than heeding our body's natural call to rest we're likely to grab a coffee or tea, nibble a sweet snack, exercise or find some other way of powering through and pepping back up, stressing our bodies further. These days, if we do manage to rest, we are often still watching screens, reading, clicking, flicking or scrolling. The practices in Step 2 offer a powerful alternative, and a more optimal way to use a quick afternoon rest time.

Your sleep by age and stage

Your sleep changes depending on your stage of life: if you know what to expect, you might feel less anxious about natural variations across your lifetime.

Infancy

Babies enter REM sleep before non-REM sleep, and have much shorter sleep cycles than adults, and because of their small stomachs, tiny digestive tracts and large demand for food to fuel their growth, they wake to feed very frequently. Their sleep cycles are well out of sync with adult demands, which can make life very trying for parents. At about 3–4 months old, babies begin to make melatonin, which starts to give them a more defined, longer stretch of sleep. If you're the parent of a new baby, it's essential to have some simple, quick, restorative body-and-brain resting techniques at your fingertips. You'll find these on pages 107.

The sleep cycle

Throughout the night, you cycle between REM (Rapid Eye Movement) and non-REM sleep. When you fall asleep, you enter a phase of non-REM sleep, followed by a shorter period of REM sleep, and so on. There are three stages to non-REM sleep. In the first, your eyes are closed but you are easily awakened. In the second, you are sleeping lightly but your body temperature is dropping and your heart rate is slowing in preparation for the third (blissful) stage, deep sleep. In this stage, your body does all the clever stuff of repairing and regenerating tissues, building bone and muscle and boosting your immune system. You then move into REM sleep, often called active sleep or paradoxical sleep, as your brain is most active and this is typically the phase in which you dream. The first REM phase lasts for 10 minutes or so and when you come into REM each time, it lasts longer, with the longest you'll stay there about an hour. REM sleep accounts for about 20 per cent of adults' sleep, but up to 50 per cent of babies' sleep.

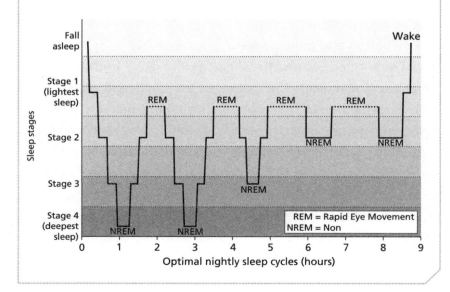

Adolescence

If you're a teenager, you are not just trying to be difficult by going to sleep late and sleeping well into the day. For many teens, the sleep phase occurs towards the late side, which means you may naturally find it easier to stay up later and harder to wake early in the morning. We produce more melatonin in our teen years than at any other time, so it's not surprising that you tend to sleep a lot: the development that establishes the adult body and brain takes place at this time.

Adulthood

If you're post-teenage and pre-elder, you'll probably see a levelling out of your average sleeping patterns, and the eight-hour average is just that – many people healthily sleep a bit less or a bit more, between seven and nine hours, and this can fluctuate from day to day and week to week, much like your appetite for food.

> ## How much of your time do you spend asleep?
>
> Babies: 66.7% = 16 hours
> Adults: 33.3% = 8 hours
> Elders: 23.0% = 5.5 hours

Menstruation and menopause

If you're a woman at menstrual age, you're likely to have a harder time sleeping during the premenstrual time and during your menstrual period, as the hormonal shifts will increase your core body temperature and trick your body into feeling more wakeful as a result. If you're experiencing peri-menopause or menopause, the hormonal fluctuations that increase your body temperature can interrupt your sleep. It's especially useful to avoid sugar and alcohol at this time because they can worsen fluctuations in hormones and spike your body heat.

Older age

Although there is always variation, as we get older – from 60 onwards – we're biologically more likely to want to go to sleep earlier and wake earlier, and will likely sleep less. Our melatonin production will decrease to about a quarter of the amount we had in young adulthood, which means getting to sleep and staying asleep can be a slightly more delicate process. A diet rich in tryptophan may be helpful. It's also worth knowing that daily exercise can be helpful in promoting deeper sleep, and that resting for short periods during the day is normal.

The temperature effect

Throughout the day, even without you realising it, your body temperature will fluctuate in line with natural circadian rhythms. If all is working normally, your core body temperature will dip at around 9 to 10 p.m. – after dark and before bedtime, depending on the season. If you had an intense workout, spent time in a sauna or had an overly hot bath or shower during this time, the rise in core body temperature might throw off your body's internal thermostat, tricking your body into waking up. If you do any of these things, notice the effect and record it in your personal sleep tracker. For most people, it's good sense to sleep in a bedroom that is as cool as possible without becoming cold, supporting the temperature cues towards sleep. While your core body temperature needs to drop, it's also a good idea to keep your extremities warm, especially your feet. Sleep socks may not be sexy, but they can help you to tolerate sleeping in a colder room without becoming too chilled.

A play of the light

I live in the UK, and during half the year there is very little daylight, both because of its northern latitude and because of the grey, rainy weather. If I stay inside all day and don't make a conscious effort to take in some sunshine (if there is any), I can feel my mood dip and I can't get to sleep easily. A lack of daylight throws off the natural mechanisms in the brain that use light and dark to determine waking and sleeping hours. Bright daylight is a part of the blue light spectrum, which specifically triggers the daytime brain response. Electronic screens, LED and fluorescent lights emit blue spectrum light that mimics daylight. If we're exposed to these at night, they work against our ability to sleep, making us feel more awake.

According to one theory, blue-light exposure late at night can trick your brain into responding with anti-sleep cues, inhibiting the production of melatonin. Other research seems to indicate that the jury is still out. 'Red' light from candlelight or soft incandescent bulbs does not have the same daylight effect, which is the rationale behind the sepia-toned night-time modes on new electronics.

Light at night can interfere with your sleep: in cities, ambient light pollution – the shine from street lights or other people's homes – can trick your brain into turning night into day. If you're a sensitive sleeper, you may wake naturally as the outside environment inches towards daylight. Keeping your bedroom dark with blackout blinds or curtains, a full shade that seals around your window completely, or wearing a well-fitting opaque eye mask, can be very helpful in keeping you asleep.

DON'T BE SAD: SEASONAL DOWNS

If you're not getting enough daylight exposure during the autumn/ winter months, this can cause a phenomenon called Seasonal Affective Disorder (SAD). If you find your energy is very low and you tend towards depressive symptoms in the winter months, your

Screen time

Using phones, tablets and computers at night may sabotage our sleep because screens emit blue light, which the eyes register as a daytime cue. Also, interacting with devices involves heightened mental activity and brainwave patterns (see Step 3) that are appropriate for the most active wake time. By being on our smartphones or computers, we maintain a high level of mental activity right up till sleep time, which is counterproductive for creating the body and brain cues for relaxation and rest. It's best to put away your phone or computer an hour or more before going to sleep. Use the Simple Sleep Sequence on page 42 to calm your body and mind, and if you're still not sleepy, read a (real, paper) book.

- Turn screens to the lowest brightness setting in the evening / night-time. Many new devices have dimmer or 'warm light' options.
- Begin turning down lights in the home an hour before bedtime if possible. Dimmer switches or low-light lamps are a helpful addition to your home as an alternative to bright overhead lights.
- Finish online or phone interactions, especially high-intensity conversations, an hour before bed so you become present in your surroundings and can settle mentally and emotionally.
- Avoiding screen time an hour or more before bed allows the serotonin to melatonin conversion.
- Keep light-emitting devices as far from your eyes as possible, and cut down the use of phone screens, computers, tablets and even television screens, as they all emit light.
- Use a non-ticking clock rather than a smartphone in your bedroom if you need a wake-up alarm.
- Read printed materials, rather than screens, using warm light at night.
- Keep social media, work and other distractions out of the bedroom.
- If you're in a one-room apartment or a hotel room, place all electronics in a drawer or closet before bed, or at least cover them with a blanket, creating a separation from work and interactions and allowing a 'contained' space for sleep.

SAD tips

- Get out into the daylight for a walk as much as possible, and – without staring into the sun – do turn your eyes skyward.
- Take exercise in the morning to boost your endorphins – higher intensity workouts earlier in the day will leave you feeling refreshed. Running or an aerobic or interval-training workout can boost the feel-good brain chemistry.
- Vitamin D is essential – in some climates with low light in winter, it's useful to take a supplement. An oral spray can be a great way to deliver the vitamin directly and effectively. Do check with your healthcare practitioner first.
- Use a bright light lamp during the first few hours of the day, boosting your exposure to what your body 'reads' as sunlight.

problems with sleep may be part of this general set of issues. You might find that taking care to get into the natural sunlight as much as possible – sitting by a window, taking a morning walk, and turning your eyes skyward – helps you to cope and resets your sleep–wake clock. If you can't get natural sunlight, using a blue-spectrum bright light lamp in the morning can be a powerful way to help keep your body clock set to a reasonable sleep–wake pattern.

DARK NIGHTS, BRIGHT MORNINGS

Light Therapy can complement your Sleep Recovery. According to the US-based Mayo Clinic, light-box therapy can help with SAD, non-seasonal depression, jet lag, sleep disorders, and adjusting to a night-time work schedule. The intensity, duration and timing of bright light/light box use is essential. First, the lux (amount of light received) needs to be 10,000-lux held at 40–60 centimetres (16–24 inches) from your face for about 20 to 30 minutes early in the morning, after you first wake up. Light should enter your eyes indirectly to prevent eye damage, and it's recommended that you consult a physician about the intensity, duration and timing of light-box therapy for depression or to help with shift work or SAD. I've used mine for mild seasonal blues and to help with jet lag, placing it on my breakfast table for 20 minutes in the morning, and it seems to have helped my mood and energy levels.

If you feel you regularly wake too early, it's worth knowing that many of us go to bed far too late for our natural wake time, which can be initiated by the breaking of dawn. If you think your problem is *waking too early*, it may be that your wake time is actually fine: it's more likely that your going-to-sleep time is the problem! The key here is not to fight the early wake time, but to plan your sleep time around it to the greatest extent possible by going to bed at a time that enables you to get the sleep hours you need. If you follow the natural rhythms, you'll find your sleep gets on track far more easily, as you're essentially no longer swimming upstream.

TURNING NIGHT INTO DAY

Changing your sleep and wake times as required by shift work can be a recipe for sleep disaster. Doctors, nurses, flight crew, police, firefighters and others with round-the-clock occupations can suffer the most from the effects of shift work as they have to change their working hours often on a weekly or monthly basis, which can result in very disjointed sleep patterns if the body doesn't adjust easily. If you work a purely nocturnal job (club DJ, night taxi driver, night-watch guard etc), you can suffer major sleep disruptions as well, because sleep quality is affected not just by the number of hours you sleep but also by the time of day in which the sleep occurs, because of ambient light and darkness. Working against millions of years of human evolution to try to reorganise your sleep–wake patterns can be a losing proposition – and some people are more sensitive than others – but overleaf are some tips that can help.

Shift work remedies

While it's easier for some people than for others, research suggests that you can better adjust to shift work over time by managing light and darkness exposure.

A study involving a group of nurses working night shifts in Quebec, Canada, had half the nurses go about their work and home life as usual and the other half were exposed intermittently to bright, full-spectrum white light, which includes the bright morning blue spectrum light, for the first six hours of their shifts. They were also asked to wear dark glasses while travelling home and, once they got there, to keep their environment dark for eight hours. They fared better than their counterparts who didn't 'turn night into day' as completely. Hormones including melatonin and cortisol, as well as their body temperatures, adjusted to the shift in their sleep/wake times more fully when they managed light and dark in ways that signalled 'day' during their night shift and 'night' during their trip home and for eight hours thereafter.

- Remain in darkness for eight hours after a shift to allow your body to create the hormones you need for good sleep.
- Exposure to bright full spectrum white light during the first six hours of your working shift can help you remain alert.
- Make sure you have the nutritional support needed to create the serotonin that converts to melatonin, making you sleepy. Foods like oats, bananas and turkey contain tryptophan, from which serotonin is created. If melatonin is available where you live, you may ask a doctor or naturopath if this would be recommended for you, especially for the first nights of a new shift pattern.
- Use the Simple Sleep Sequence after work (page 42) and before bed, as well as practices like the Breath of Joy (page 103) just after your wake time. Avoid caffeine in favour of stimulating breath practices if you need extra energy.
- Eating a healthy, balanced diet can be more difficult when wholesome food is less accessible during the night-time hours. On your off days, make healthy meals with enough vegetables and protein to nourish you and bring them to work with you or pre-order healthy meals from a delivery service.

JET LAG

When you've taken a flight through different time zones, the disjoint between where you are now and where you were previously leads to the set of symptoms we call 'jet lag'. Your body isn't able to align day and night light cues with what it expects, and even the climate may be different. It is natural that it can take some time to adjust, making the right hormones to correspond with the time of day. The general rule is a day for every hour difference in time zone to reset. If you can align your sunlight exposure and eating times to the local time zone before you travel, this can help you adjust more easily to the new time when you land.

Jet lag remedies

* Set your watch to your destination time as soon as you get on the plane. Eat and sleep on the schedule of your destination if you can.
* Get some sunlight when you first arrive at your destination and stay up until a reasonable bedtime for your location.
* Avoid alcohol on the plane if possible – you may be able to sleep on the plane after a drink or two but the quality of your sleep will be lower if under the influence.
* If you choose to take a nap on your day of arrival, make sure that it is as short as you can manage.
* In some countries, melatonin in pill form is available – if you choose to use this, it is only really effective for the first night or two, so be careful not to overuse it, and take it in consultation with a qualified naturopath or doctor.
* Use wake-up (page 77) and power-down practices (see page 91) to help you manage your energy without resorting to (excessive or ill-timed) caffeine use.

Energy on credit: caffeine, adenosine, adrenaline

If you're tired from a lack of sleep, it's really important to know that there's a big difference between real, sustainable energy that comes from nutrition and rest, and the kind of false energy that is borrowed from your body's reserves, or is generated by stress.

In Step 2, we'll talk more about this distinction, which one of my colleagues described to me as 'like borrowing from the energy credit card instead of taking money out of the energy bank'. Caffeine is one way that many people take energy on credit. Let's look at how this happens, so you can use your credit wisely and build up the energy funds in the bank.

Caffeine is one of the most popular and readily available stimulants. It's also one of the most addictive, because it gets involved with a cocktail of three powerful brain chemicals, making caffeine feel, temporarily, like a good solution to a bad night's sleep. But if you use too much, too frequently, caffeine can break down some of the natural reactions your body relies on to get you to sleep.

One of the main things that caffeine does is trick your brain into thinking you're less tired than you actually are. A chemical called adenosine builds up in your brain when you're tired, which tells your central nervous system that you need rest. When adenosine connects with its specific receptors in your brain, the brain slows down its activity, which makes you feel sleepy, and your blood vessels dilate (expand) for good oxygen flow during sleep. Caffeine effectively pushes into the places where the adenosine molecules are meant to bring the sleepiness message. The caffeine binds to its same receptors and lets fewer of them soak up the tiredness cues to slow down and sleep or rest: the natural slowing-down signals don't fire. Instead, your brain activity actually speeds up. Basically, caffeine tricks your brain into thinking you don't need rest when you really do!

Your morning coffee also pings your pituitary gland to release hormones that spark your adrenal glands to make adrenaline – the 'fight or flight' hormone. When you're under threat or stress, adrenaline boosts your alertness: you snap to attention more sharply, and get a burst of energy to mobilise against a threat. Interestingly, although caffeine doesn't create the kind of tolerance that makes you seek increasing amounts to get the same hit, you do very quickly become physically dependent upon the jolt it gives, partly because of a third chemical that's involved: dopamine.

Dopamine is the same feel-good neurotransmitter involved in addictive drugs like cocaine. Caffeine delivers dopamine into your brain's feel-good pleasure circuits and its very more-ish quality makes it a tough habit to kick. I notice on caffeine-free yoga retreats that about half the participants will have a caffeine withdrawal headache on the first day or two, and some people feel excessively sleepy and/or a bit queasy or nauseated.

Ollie had no idea that the same afternoon coffee that powered him for his long runs after work was keeping him awake at night. When he stopped drinking coffee before working out, and instead did a brief meditation before getting his running shoes on, he found his sleep improved dramatically.

My friend Susanne regularly has a cup of coffee after a late meal, or a cup of strong tea in the late afternoon, and has no trouble getting to sleep. I envy her ability to have a nice espresso after dinner. While this is not altogether uncommon, if you're like most people with delicate sleep and a more highly strung nervous system, or a more pronounced chemical sensitivity to caffeine, your coffee or tea can affect you for hours after you get the initial effect.

Caffeine has an average half-life of two and a half to six hours. I use four hours as a general guide, which means that, depending on your metabolism, only about half the caffeine of your double espresso or extra-large English breakfast tea is metabolised out of your system *four to six hours after you drink it.* Have a look at the chart (below) to check out the content of your caffeine fix. Choosing options that lower your caffeine intake, especially later in the day, can help you minimise your dependency on it or sidestep the sleep-sabotaging effects of your daily cup.

I hate to break bad news to you, but if you enjoy chocolate with a high cocoa content, it's worth knowing that it contains caffeine and theobromine, both of which have stimulant effects. Notice the effect that chocolate may have on you if you eat it later in the day or at night. A cup of night-time cocoa with a high chocolate content may soothe your soul, but may also stimulate your nervous

The caffeine half-life

I f you drink a double espresso at 8 a.m., it's only half gone at noon, given average caffeine metabolism. At 4 p.m., one-quarter of it is probably still kicking around in your system. An eighth of your double espresso is still there at 8 p.m. and finally, by midnight, there are just traces left. Now, if you have that same double espresso at 4 p.m., a single espresso is still buzzing around at 8 p.m., and half an espresso is still in your system at midnight.

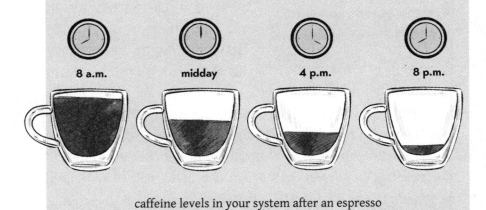

| 8 a.m. | midday | 4 p.m. | 8 p.m. |

caffeine levels in your system after an espresso

Liz stopped getting a 3 p.m. latte from the coffee shop on the corner or a filter coffee from the office kitchen and instead took a mid-afternoon rest in the elevated leg position described in Step 2 (page 115). For her, it worked wonders. This is because resting decreases the neurotransmitter adenosine – the one that tells your body you're tired and need rest. Taking a short, effective rest like those described makes you less tired, less stressed, and healthier overall. These poses help you avoid the need for caffeine in the afternoon, and they help to recondition your nervous system so you have healthy energy levels all day, and can fall asleep more easily and deeply at night.

system. For this reason, many people are now experimenting with mixes of calming spices before bed, such as cinnamon, turmeric and cardamom.

Knowledge is power – and while I'm not saying you must give up your morning coffee, it's important that you understand the trade-offs involved in using caffeine and that you track your sensitivity to it.

If you do give up caffeine entirely, after an initial withdrawal period – which can involve pretty gnarly headaches and irritability – I've noticed in myself and in my clients a definite *decrease* in tension, visible in a calmer face, less tension in the muscles and an increase in ease and relaxation. This generally translates quickly into getting to sleep or staying asleep more easily.

HOW MUCH CAFFEINE?

The table overleaf shows the broad span of caffeine content found in your cup of coffee or tea (including decaffeinated), your soft drink or your mug of cocoa. If you regularly drink bottled beverages, it's worth knowing how much of a jolt you're getting: the caffeine content can be found online at sites like caffeineinformer.com.

Caffeine content in common beverages

Coffee drinks	Size in oz. (ml)	Caffeine (mg)
Brewed	8 (237)	95-165
Latte or mocha	8 (237)	63-126
Instant	8 (237)	63
Americano espresso	12 (360)	154
Espresso	1 (30)	47-64
Brewed, decaf	8 (237)	2-5
Instant, decaf	8 (237)	2
Espresso, decaf	1 (30)	0

Teas	Size in oz. (ml)	Caffeine (mg)
Brewed black	8 (237)	25-48
Ready-to-drink, bottled black	8 (237)	5-40
Brewed green	8 (237)	25-29
Brewed black, decaf	8 (237)	2-5
Matcha	8 (237)	70

Soft drinks	Size in oz. (ml)	Caffeine (mg)
Cola	8 (237)	24-46
Citrus (most brands)	8 (237)	0
Root beer (most brands)	8 (237)	0

Energy drinks	Size in oz. (ml)	Caffeine (mg)
Energy drink	8 (237)	27-164
Energy shot	1 (30)	40-100

Chocolate drinks	Size in oz. (ml)	Caffeine (mg)
Hot Chocolate (powdered mix)	8 (237)	5
Cacao (nibs or raw powdered form)	1 (30)	22

INSTEAD OF CAFFEINE:
ENERGISING FULL-BODY WAKE-UP

Too little – or unsatisfying – sleep will leave us feeling tired in the morning. It may seem counter-intuitive, but one of the best methods for dealing with morning exhaustion is not to try to get a few extra minutes of sleep, but to get out of bed and do some simple body movements to improve your focus, activating your body-to-brain wake-up cues. These will help you to start your day feeling more focused and clear-headed. In general, they make more space so you can breathe deeply, elevate your heart rate, freshen your face, activate the muscles in your legs and get your feet firmly planted on the ground.

Energising full-body wake-up: The exercises

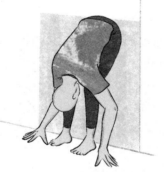

1 Wall-backed Forward Bend

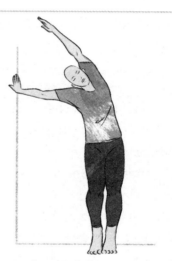

2 Wide-armed Chest Stretch

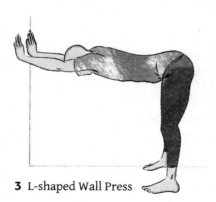

3 L-shaped Wall Press

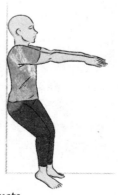

4 Wall Squats

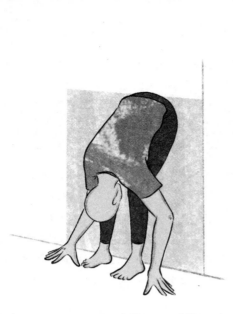

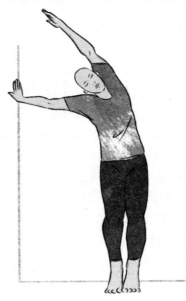

1 Wall-backed Forward Bend

With your back to the wall, fold forwards with your knees bent deeply, so that your chest rests on or between your thighs. Breathe in and out evenly, lengthening your inhalation slightly. This improves circulation into your chest, flushes your face and releases your neck and the long muscles that line your spine.

2 Wide-armed Chest Stretch

Stand sideways-on to a wall and place the palm of the nearest hand to the wall, with the arm stretched straight. Lift the other arm up and over your head towards the wall, taking long, deep inhalations and settling your shoulders, especially on your exhalation. This stretches the intercostal muscles between your ribs, freeing up your breath and making you feel more spacious.

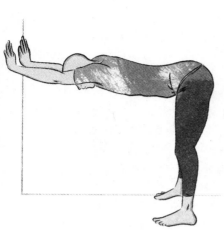

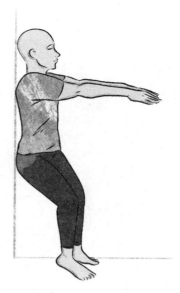

3 L-shaped Wall Press

4 Wall Squats

Stand facing the wall, bend forwards and place your hands wider than shoulder-width apart, at hip height. You'll make an upside-down L shape with your body. Breathe deeply, lengthening your hips back, swaying from side to side to loosen the muscles that line your spine. For more circulation and energy in your arms, bend your elbows and press back a few times, doing a form of wall push-up.

With your back to the wall, bend your knees, sliding down the wall. Extend your arms out directly in front of you, palms level with your shoulders and facing down. Hold for between two and five breaths. Lift your arms up over your head to make it more energising. These wall squats power up your legs and leave you feeling steady.

5 Breath of Joy
For an energy burst at the end of this practice, add the Breath of Joy sequence (see page 103).

Tea and sympathy

In the UK, where I live, a cup of tea is soothing for the soul. It's associated with comfort – the phrase 'tea and sympathy' is one that conjures up an image of a cuppa and a chat with a loved one or friend. However, the caffeine in what the British call *normal* tea may provide a boost and a lift to the mood, but it can interfere with sleep if taken too late in the day. Before bed and in the hours before sleeping, given how long it takes for caffeine to leave your system, it's best to avoid coffee – according to some sources, even decaf can have a small amount of caffeine that affects some people – as well as black tea, green tea, white tea, matcha, guarana, taurine energy drinks or snacks and or chocolate/cacao drinks. They all contain some amount of caffeine or stimulant (see page 76).

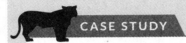

CASE STUDY

Liz was regularly sitting down with a cup of black tea and a book before bed, not realising that even though she could fall asleep okay, the caffeine was disturbing her sleep by making her more likely to wake in the middle of the night, after her deepest exhaustion had worn off and her nervous system was more susceptible to waking. I recommended that she try a good-quality herbal chamomile tea, or an infusion of lemon balm or French vervain. She tried my favourites, a sleep blend made by Pukka Herbs in the UK, and a brilliant tea called Bengal Spice by Celestial Seasonings, made in the US. She kept those to hand as well as Rooibos (red bush), a South African favourite with a taste somewhat similar to black tea but which contains no caffeine.

Warm milk and soothing spices

Heat a mugful of dairy milk or plant milk (almond, soy, etc) in a saucepan over low heat. Both dairy milk and soy/soya milk are noted to contain tryptophan, which can contribute to the production of serotonin and melatonin.

Whisk in while heating the milk:

* ½ teaspoon turmeric powder, known for its anti-inflammatory properties and to soothe digestion. Use a stainless-steel saucepan as turmeric can stain enamel.
* ¼ teaspoon of cinnamon
* 1 cardamom pod – split open the pod with the handle of a knife and put it in the milk whole or grind the seeds. Cardamom powder is okay but less potent.
* A few black peppercorns, for heat, and to enhance absorption of the anti-inflammatory and soothing curcumin in the turmeric
* 1 arm of star anise – a little goes a long way

Turn off the heat just before the milk boils.

* If you're using dairy milk and a skin forms on the top, this is normal – just skim it off and then pour the mixture into a cup. Let the peppercorns, star anise and cardamom settle to the bottom or strain them out with a fine sieve or tea strainer.
* You can add a small amount of honey or sweetener if desired, but be careful not to take so much that you create a sugar spike. This can be counterproductive when you're trying to get to sleep.

Pour into your favourite mug, sip slowly and enjoy with low lighting... then brush your teeth and prepare for bed with the Simple Sleep Sequence on page 42.

Tip: For a simple snack to go with your drink, two or three plain oatcakes or oat biscuits can boost your tryptophan levels, and since oats have a low glycemic index, they can be sustaining and prevent before-bed munchies.

THE ALCOHOL EFFECT

You may be tempted to have a late-night drink to calm your nerves before bed, but while this may soothe you in the short term, your nightcap may prove counterproductive just a couple of hours later. This is why: when you down a glass of whisky or wine, it passes through your digestive tract, where it gets whisked into your blood vessels, and your blood then shunts it around to all parts of your body – including your brain. Alcohol affects several brain chemicals, including gamma-Aminobutyric acid (GABA), which plays a role in calming you by making certain neurons less excitable. This spike in GABA accounts for the initial relaxing effect of your drink. Alcohol binds to the GABA receptor, and trips off reactions that slow down the activity in your brain activity further, giving you a soothing, sedating effect. Alcohol also reduces the effect of an excitatory neurotransmitter called glutamate and helps to increase the release of dopamine (the feel-good happy hormone).

Because GABA inhibits or slows down certain 'excitatory impulses' in your brain, you may get an initial anti-anxiety and calming effect, but as your brain's chemistry readjusts, you're likely to be left with a bounce-back effect that can wake you in the middle of the night with your heart beating faster, sweaty sheets or nightclothes, and anxious thoughts. Since alcohol is mostly sugar, when it's broken down by your liver it causes your body temperature to rise and gives you a sugar spike, which also disturbs your sleep. Cutting out or keeping alcohol to a bare minimum, and having it long before bedtime, can go a long way to rebuilding natural and truly restful sleep.

STEP 2

Replenish your energy

If your nervous system is constantly buzzing, you may be extremely stressed, or you might be so accustomed to the heightened state that it just feels normal. Either way, we can be under so much subtle pressure to perform, to power through and to keep going, that we draw upon energy reserves rather than being truly resourced. In this second Sleep Recovery step, you will learn important skills that will enable you to move from the over-stimulated fight-flight response to the rest-and-digest calm state that puts energy back on the grid. You'll learn what you can do each day to soothe your jangled nerves and get some good sleep.

In **Part 1** of this Sleep Recovery step, you'll discover how to unhook the chronic stress response that has so many of us sleeping poorly. You'll use the innate features of your nervous system to get you out of the stress response and into a calmer state that repairs your rest. You'll begin with easy breathing practices and with decreasing tension in your body so that you can settle into the more powerful breathing practices. When you breathe easily and fully, and use some basic techniques, you will heal your nervous system and your sleep will follow.

While of course you're aware that breath is essential to life, you may not know how profoundly *changing your breathing* changes your body and your brain chemistry, your mindset and your emotional state. Breathing is one of our most deeply ingrained response mechanisms, and when we learn how to harness its power, we can easily soothe our jangled nervous systems to get to sleep, rest more deeply and feel better all day.

Before I began to practise yoga, I could barely breathe, my body wouldn't settle, and my mind would spin out, so I know breathing practices can be hard to do before you settle your body a bit. Once I started doing yoga, I quickly saw that I had unconsciously developed the bad habit of breathing as shallowly and quickly as possible. Breathing makes space and gives life, and not breathing well, whatever the cause, gets in the way of sleeping well.

Part 2 involves repairing your body's innate relaxation response by using Restorative yoga poses. If you haven't heard of these before, they involve placing your body in intentional, supported relaxed positions: allowing the body to be supported by cushions, blankets or other props creates a sense of deep release. Essentially a form of conscious lounging, these poses provide a much-needed pause for your body, mind and soul to come back into balance throughout the day. They work by shifting your circulation in ways that are seen as benefitting different organs. Rest positions can be used by almost everyone; each creates a different effect and feeling. While I suggest practising all of them, I'll also show you how each pose of the three recommended restoratives may particularly suit each of the three sleep personalities.

These tools have helped me and also the people you'll meet in this chapter to get to sleep, to stay asleep or to feel more alert during the day.

PART 1:
SHIFT FROM FIGHT OR FLIGHT
TO REST AND DIGEST

ALL HUMAN BEINGS, when under threat, tighten up, and take up less space and use less oxygen. When we are happy and safe, we expand: our muscles relax, we breathe more easily and deeply. Most of the threats we face are no longer immediate physical danger – we don't often have to run from wild animals – but instead we feel unsafe when disasters happen: we get divorced, or a friend dies in a car crash; we're diagnosed with a tumour, lose our livelihood, or come home to a house that's been broken into. Our bodies harden in response and we inure ourselves to further pain. When we batten down the hatches, our breathing tightens up. If we breathe we will *feel more*, and feeling isn't fun at times like these. The activation response causes our limbs to lose blood flow and tighten against the bone. Our bodies evolved to do this, so that if we are cut in a dangerous situation, we don't bleed out. Breathing only just enough when we're in peril dulls our sensation, and can at first protect us from overwhelm.

The paradox is that most of the time we're not under mortal threat: if we breathe and dismantle the body armour, the pain can rise to the surface, we'll feel it, and mostly, the fear and pain will not kill us. If we breathe, we feel, and the feeling moves through.

People with sleep apnoea wake in the night many times; in some of the worst cases, several times per minute. If your airway is blocked, your body sends an alarm call to your brain to jolt you awake enough to draw breath again. We are elegantly designed that way, in order to keep us alive. Breathing is survival, so the breath-to-brain response system is powerful and direct.

Your body-brain-mind-emotion response systems affect your sleep and the quality of your life. Some basic knowledge and simple practice will give you tremendous power to change your mind and mood, and over time you can recondition and repair your sleep and become fundamentally calmer, less depressed or anxious, and just plain happier. Later in this chapter I will tell you a story about when I learned to breathe in a way that gave me a very different way of opening up.

How it works

You have a central nervous system made up of the brain and spinal cord and one branch, called the *peripheral* nervous system, that links the central one to the periphery – the stuff outside the brain and spinal cord – to the other bits: the organs, muscles, bones and viscera. This messaging system relays messages from body-to-brain and brain-to-body, with the somatic (body-related) aspect involving both motor (movement-related) and sensory messengers.

The other branch, called the *autonomic* nervous system, works on activating and relaxing responses throughout your body, adjusting your body's reactions to maintain constant balance in the nervous system, responding to the environment appropriately by changing your heart rate, stimulating or decreasing, speeding up or slowing down your

The nervous system

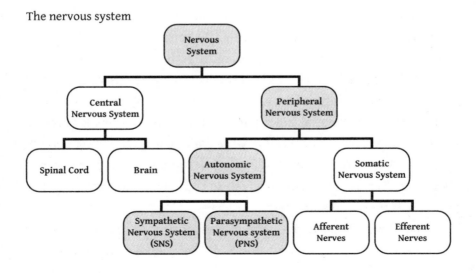

breathing and controlling salivation, sweating, sexual arousal, having to pee, as well as the blood flow to your muscles and organs.

This system of messaging involves feedback loops that bring sensory information from the external environment and from your body's internal sense back to the brain, where it can be quickly processed by different parts of the brain, and changes can be mobilised. If you're in danger, your body sense will pick up on it, and transmit sense information to your brain, which does things like spike your blood pressure and release the stress hormones you'd need to make a quick getaway.

If all works well, this response system goes about its business quietly and unnoticed, but interestingly, this is one of the keys to affecting our brain, our hormones, and our sense of well-being through what we do with our bodies. Because we have partial control over this alarm and deactivation system, we can do lots of things that lower our stress levels, help us to sleep well, and feel generally better and more easeful.

Every day you'll go back and forth between activation and relaxation. The sympathetic nervous system (SNS) is the part that 'activates' and the parasympathetic nervous system (PNS) is the part that 'relaxes'. When one is heightened, the other deactivates. The one that's dominant depends on what's happening inside you and what's happening in your environment.

The autonomic nervous system see-saw

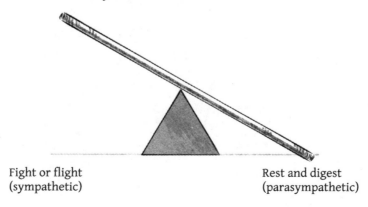

Fight or flight
(sympathetic)

Rest and digest
(parasympathetic)

SYMPATHETIC NERVOUS SYSTEM: ACTIVATING, FIGHT OR FLIGHT

If we call it 'fight or flight', we might get the wrong idea about the sympathetic nervous system: that identifies what it does at the extreme end of the spectrum. You need the activation part of your nervous system to get up and do things – go for a run, learn new things, meet pressured deadlines, chase after children to stop them running into the street. It activates both brain and body, mobilising

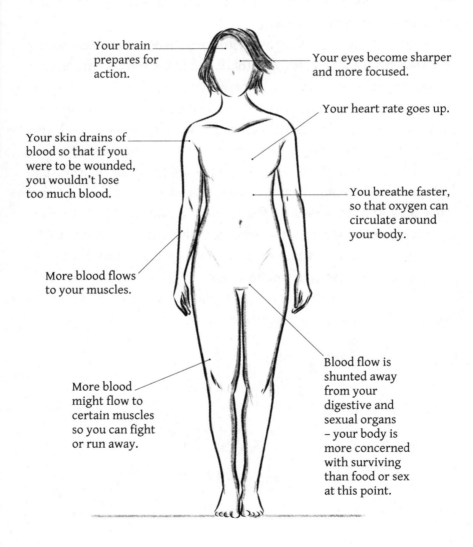

Your brain prepares for action.

Your eyes become sharper and more focused.

Your heart rate goes up.

Your skin drains of blood so that if you were to be wounded, you wouldn't lose too much blood.

You breathe faster, so that oxygen can circulate around your body.

More blood flows to your muscles.

More blood might flow to certain muscles so you can fight or run away.

Blood flow is shunted away from your digestive and sexual organs – your body is more concerned with surviving than food or sex at this point.

it for action. When you're under stress, fearful or over-agitated, this sympathetic nervous system revs up into fight, flight, freeze and other extreme reactions. All of these things happen when you're in activation mode: (see figure opposite).

In full-blown response mode, you will feel totally focused on the thing that's incited the reaction. Because this is, at its extreme, survival mode, it uses your resources – and even your reserves.

This system evolved far earlier than the prefrontal cortex (the logical thought part) of our brains, so it's not too well attuned to the circumstances of our modern lives. Yours will activate when you find something threatening, even though it doesn't require you to run away or fight. The more threatened and fearful we feel, the more this system kicks into gear. Evolutionarily, human beings that had sensitive activation systems were quick to get away from danger. But now a heightened SNS just makes us stressy and fraught. In fact, chronic over-activation can leave your body and mind exhausted as it uses up energy and depletes your body's resources, making life more difficult because our modern problems require level-headedness and diplomacy more than fast legs or fists. But still we amp up in response to stress, and when the stress hormones flood your body, you're often trapped without the ability to discharge all the extra energy that's available. This is where exercise, yoga and breath practices can provide a vital resource for letting off steam, but also help to down-regulate your nervous system so that you're not so tightly wound, and the hair trigger is dismantled. A calmer system overall enables a right-sized response to stress or perceived threat and the ability to dissipate the stress hormones.

Some of the practices in this step, including the breathing practices on page 92, are useful to help you energise when you need to spark your sympathetic nervous system slightly, without stressing your body. I recommend these for a sustainable morning wake-up, and as an afternoon pick-me-up once you've had a bit of rest. They help you to feel brighter without a caffeine or sugar hit.

PARASYMPATHETIC NERVOUS SYSTEM: RELAXING, REST AND DIGEST

On the other side of the spectrum sits the 'rest and digest' part of the system. It's active when you're calmly lounging and reading this book, during most of your time asleep and when you're drowsy after a big meal. This part of the system slows down your heart rate and stimulates your immune system.

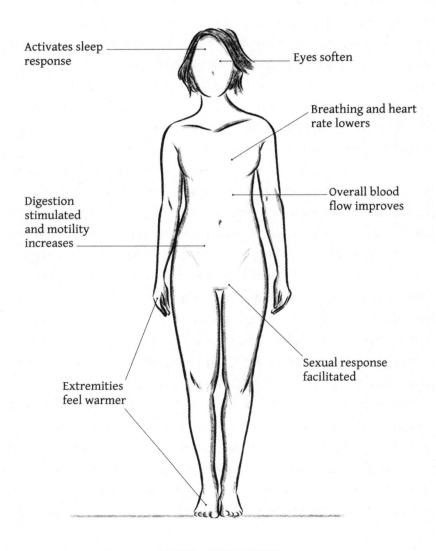

Activates sleep response

Eyes soften

Breathing and heart rate lowers

Overall blood flow improves

Digestion stimulated and motility increases

Sexual response facilitated

Extremities feel warmer

Activating the parasympathetic nervous system gets blood flow going all over your body more generally. This is why when you're more relaxed, your hands and feet feel less cold. By bringing more circulation to your digestive tract, it stimulates digestion. This helps to build your body's resources. While this should be our state when we're at rest, as a society we may be seeing a shift towards a higher base level of arousal in our nervous systems. We are living at a faster pace, we are more reliant on stimulants, we're more inundated with information, light, noise, and all-hour alertness than in any generation before. If we are in sympathetic mode too much of the time, it's no wonder that so many of us are fatigued and depleted. At the same time, when hyper-stimulation is the cause of the exhaustion, that makes it all the more difficult to drop into the relaxed (parasympathetic) state we need in order to feel really restored.

Relearn how to (really) relax

In order to recondition your capacity to sleep, you need to redevelop the ability to relax fully, not just at bedtime but throughout the day. Herbert Benson, a cardiologist at Harvard Medical School and a pioneer in the field of mind–body medicine, found that the body can enter a deep parasympathetic state where it uses less oxygen and glucose (meaning we use less energy) than at any other time, including during sleep. He termed this state the 'relaxation response'. His research shows it takes a minimum of three minutes to enter this state, although usually it's longer. For those struggling with fatigue and insomnia, it is essential to learn how to enter this state to allow the body to recalibrate and start conserving and rebuilding resources that are depleted when sleep is poor or lacking.

I explain this process to my clients as 'putting energy back on the grid' when we are tired. Spending time moving into the relaxation response retrains the body and brain in the states needed to move towards sleep, and to stay asleep.

One of the most important things you can learn, to help you repair your ability to rest, is to breathe in a way that balances and calms you.

BREATHE FOR BALANCE, TO ENERGISE OR TO RELAX

This basic practice involves breathing in and out for the same duration, called sama-vritti (Sanskrit, meaning 'same wave'), and balances the activating and relaxing aspects of your nervous system.

Your breath works in mysterious and fascinating ways. For example, lengthening your exhale subtly lowers your heart rate and fosters relaxation, while increasing the length of your inhalation increases your heart rate and can have a stimulating effect. Another, slightly odder fact is that your two nostrils correspond to the two aspects of the nervous system. If you breathe in and out through your right nostril (called surya bhedana or sun-piercing breath in the yoga tradition, see page 103), it has a stimulating effect on the sympathetic nervous system. Breathing in and out through your left nostril, on the other hand, known in the yoga tradition as chandra bhedana (moon-piercing breath, see page 100), has a subtle calming effect on the parasympathetic nervous system. These effects are best felt if you have no breathing difficulties – you may not feel the effects as clearly if you have asthma or a blocked nose.

HOW TO DO THE BASIC YOGA BREATH

As we saw in Step 1, this is a classic yoga-based technique for being sufficiently aware of your breath to change it. We'll call it a cleansing breath. Called ujjayii, it's referred to as the classic 'yoga breath'. If you do yoga stretches without the ujjayii breath, the postures are definitely less effective. The lengthened rhythmic breathing slows you down, sensitises you, takes the shrink-wrap off. It's the first step to then expanding and changing your breath to soothe or uplift yourself easily and sustainably. Sometimes it's useful to count *inhale*-two-three-four and *exhale* two-three-four as slowly as is comfortable, but the tempo is based on how your lungs fill and empty comfortably without too much strain.

Breathing like this makes a sound – like ocean waves in the distance. This is caused by gently constricting the back of your throat, and you can more easily focus your mind on the soft sound of your breath. When it's done with even inhalation and exhalation, it has a 'balancing' effect. When you subtly lengthen your exhale (see page 101), you slow your heart rate, which calms your nervous system and sends the message from your body to your brain that you are out of danger, you are safe. This helps you to sleep more deeply. When you want to feel more alert, you can do the opposite (see page 103) – lengthen your inhale and you'll raise your heart rate and feel more energised.

You can do this breath lying down or seated, and you can do it on its own any time. Keep this breath balanced, or add a little more time on the exhale as you do the Simple Sleep Sequence and when you begin the restorative practices at the end of this step.

- Breathe in and out through your nose only (mouth closed).
- Intentionally narrow the back of your throat to make a soft hissing or sighing sound. This streamlines and slows the flow of breath into your lungs.
- Start by inhaling normally through the nose without tightening the back of your throat.
- Exhale through your nose with the gentle tone like a sighing sound at the back of your throat.
- Once this feels easy, you can make the soft sighing sound on inhale as well as exhale.
- You can add a count to make your inhale even with your exhale.
- Keep the sound even. When you're doing it right, the sound is subtle and constant, like hearing ocean waves in the far distance.

Breathing in this way is gentle, light and smooth and does the opposite of strong, tight and staccato breathing: your body softens and relaxes.

Using this breath and directing your attention to a different part of your body brings circulation to that area, making it feel soothed and expanded. It is a general rule that where your attention goes, your circulation – what the yoga tradition calls 'prana' or life force – flows. When I teach people to breathe with awareness in their lower back area, where the kidneys sit, their eyes and face immediately soften as the body calms. I think of it as a de-adrenalising effect. This is a great tool to use throughout the day; since you can make your breath full while still quiet, no one needs to know you're directing your attention to the nourishing calming breath. I use it when I commute, in meetings, during a stressful conversation, or even in the cinema if there's a startling scene.

Space to breathe, more space to sleep

Sometimes we need reminding of the helpful things we need to do. This was the case for me even after I'd learned yoga and breath practices. There was one that I had forgotten, and I got a lucky reminder when my insomnia had resurfaced.

It was one of those 'perfect storm' times in my life – a break-up, a bereavement, a house move and a career change had brought me, and years of possessions, into a single room as a lodger. All my things were stacked in precarious piles in my room, and during a holiday party my landlady's friend approached me to ask how I was doing.

Nancy had the wild, wavy black hair streaked with white and grey, long purple layers of draped knitwear and baubles befitting someone who'd been a yoga teacher from back in the 1970s.

She asked me how the move had gone. 'Fine,' I said. 'Really well.' But the good dress and bright lipstick weren't fooling her. Nancy could see the signs of someone suffocating, and out of maternal interest she asked me if I wanted help with some decorating tips for downsizing, so I opened the door to my rented room.

'In*tense*.' She nodded at the books, suitcases, clothing, posters, stacks of photographs, sports equipment, shoes, file folders, boxes, bags. She took in a long breath and issued something between a laugh and a sigh. She waved away my attempt at an apology. 'Too much!' she said. 'You have to clear some space to be able to breathe in this place.' Nancy had hit upon the issue – I could barely breathe.

'Are you doing your full yogic breathing?' she asked. 'Of course,' I said, slightly backfooted. As a new yoga teacher I thought I knew it all, but apparently I'd forgotten or had never really been taught. 'Let me show you what I mean. It might help you get some space in there,' she said as she poked me in the ribs gently.

This is what she taught me:

First, to puff up my tummy, letting it get big like a fat Buddha, and on the exhale to relax the low abdomen. It was oddly soothing. Then she prompted me to keep doing it, but now to focus on my lower back as I breathed. It was like taking off a pair of too-tight jeans. All the tension I didn't know was there, what with all my frantic running around and party preparations, started to loosen.

Then the middle part of the ribcage. Nancy pointed to the side of her ribs, right below the bra-line, and told me to breathe just there next. 'Expand on both sides. When you get anxious your diaphragm tenses up. Breathe and open it up.' Inhaling again, she looked like a bird fluffing out its feathers. My brain didn't seem to connect up to that part of my body at first. Nancy told me to tap the sides of my ribcage to wake them up, which helped. I'd never been so precise about filling up my lungs to stretch the muscles that line the ribcage, but slowly it made sense. I'd been having mild panic attacks, and each time this area, the solar plexus, would seize up, feeling as though I was being stabbed in the stomach. Now I know that it's not an uncommon anxiety feeling. This was a way to stretch here, from the inside.

Then the upper chest. Like most people, when I was anxious I was breathing mostly in the upper front part of my chest. Nancy asked me to breathe like I could inhale into the space between my shoulder blades. It felt both calming and energising, and while my neck and shoulders tightened up when I took a breath at first, soon I learned to relax my neck and upper shoulders even as I took an inhalation. This felt great: really expansive.

I'd been practising 'yoga' for years, stretching and bending and *trying* to meditate... (more on that later) but I'd never seen anyone shunt their breath into different parts so *subtly*. I found that when I used my mind to direct the muscles and my breathing, I became conscious of what expanded and what stayed still. I added this three-part breathing into my pre-bed routine, and I felt that all the stretches I did became far more effective. As I did the breathing and paid attention to these different places as I breathed, the places seemed to light up and to *lighten* up.

Breathing like this is like clearing out the dirt: in a dark room you don't really see dirt and dust. Open the curtains, the light gets in, and the dirty corners come into focus. Similarly, when I teach this to other people they are often amazed at how tight their breathing has become through anxiety or depression, through exhaustion or simply through lack of awareness.

I used this way of breathing in the months that followed, and learned to soothe and expand myself. Life was asking me to grow bigger to accommodate all the changes, and instead of shutting down and cutting off, this new way of breathing helped me to open up. I began, and slowly my jaw unclenched, the furrow in my brow became shallower and my sleep deepened.

With this lightness and space, your overwrought, fear-sensitive nervous system can ratchet down. There will be more patience, greater sensibility, less anxiety.

HOW TO DO THREE-PART BREATH

Think of this as a space-making breath technique. You'll bring your breath into your lungs evenly, fully and calmly. To prepare for sleep, do it lying on the floor or bed with your feet on the floor and knees pointing up, with a natural arch in your lower back.

Don't press your lower back into the floor Pilates-style and don't contract your abdominals: that will inhibit the movement of the breathing muscle called the diaphragm. A relaxed curved lower-back position lets your breath move more easily into your lungs. This helps you to take the shrink-wrap off your body, to help you find balance and sanity when you need to feel safe enough to sleep.

1 Lower abdomen (low back, lower digestive tract)

* Place your hands on your lower abdomen beneath your navel, to the inside of your hip bones.
* When you breathe in, inflate your lower abdomen, relaxing the abdominal muscles to make a 'Buddha belly'. Your hands will rise.
* As you exhale, release your abdominal muscles and your hands will descend.
* Relax your lower back as you do this.
* This brings more balanced circulation to the lower back and brings circulation into the area that influences digestion.

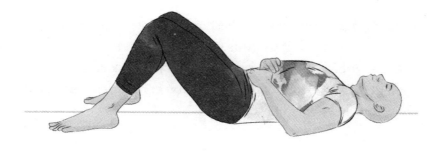

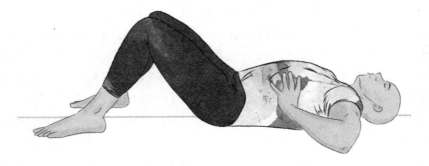

2 Middle ribcage (solar plexus, diaphragm and stomach)

◆ Wrap your fingers around the front of your ribcage, with your thumbs touching the sides of your ribs. Rest your index fingers laterally across your ribcage at the bottom of the sternum (where a bra-line would be).
◆ Keep your shoulders relaxed and elbows on the floor.
◆ As you inhale, inflate the front and back of your middle ribcage, and expand sideways at the same time.
◆ Experiment: see if you can inflate front to back then inflate side to side, and finally expand all the way around, stretching the intercostal muscles that line your ribs.
◆ As you exhale, your ribcage will naturally narrow and the muscles in between your ribs will relax.
◆ This helps expand the capacity of your lungs and improves full body circulation.

3 Upper chest (top of lungs, shoulders and neck)

◆ Place your hands on your chest, right below your collarbones, with your thumbs out towards your shoulders.
◆ As you inhale, focus your attention on the back of your shoulders, keeping them relaxed. As you exhale, release your shoulders and upper chest.

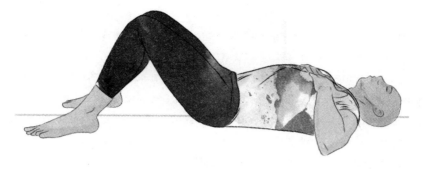

- If you try this in a mirror, you may notice that you lift your shoulders when you breathe in. De-couple your breath from pulling up your shoulders. Learn to breathe in while keeping your shoulders, neck and face relaxed.

All together: The breath wave

- Inhale and expand your lower abdomen, then your ribs, then your upper chest.
- Exhale to release the breath from the top of your chest, through the middle part of your ribs, and downwards to hollow out and soften your abdomen.
- You can use your hands to direct your attention to where you're breathing in and expanding, and where you're breathing out and softening.
- Practise so you can do this with awareness on each part separately and smoothly from bottom to top, and from top to bottom.

Repeat this several times, refining and calming your breath, keeping your face, throat and jaw relaxed. When done, lower your hands to your sides. Breathe gently and evenly through both nostrils a few times and then return to natural breath.

Find the breath count that is easy and stress-free for you. You don't want to gasp for breath or feel tightness. Keeping awareness in the back of your body as you breathe helps to enhance the grounding and relaxing effect. Using the breath wave and breath 'filling' (using the muscles to activate the areas mirroring the effect of filling a glass of water) from the bottom to the top gently keeps you from focusing your breath on the upper chest. You'll notice that some areas are easier for you to breathe into, and others are much tighter. Developing this awareness and learning to release all the areas repairs your body's sleep-readiness.

RELAXING 'LUNAR' LEFT NOSTRIL BREATHING (CHANDRA BHEDANA)

This practice draws on a physiological correspondence between the left nostril and the parasympathetic nervous system (calming) and the right nostril's correspondence with the sympathetic nervous system (stimulating). You can do this seated, but I like to do it with total support, lying down.

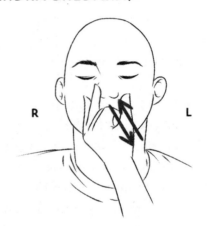

- Lie on your back in the neutral position (see page 97), with your feet on the floor or bed and your knees pointing up. You can do this with your head on a pillow if you like, but keep it low: you might find it's a bit straining if the pillow's too high.
- Place your left elbow against the same side of your ribcage and rest your left thumb gently on the place where the fleshy bit meets the bony bit of the left nostril. Your other fingers will naturally curl inward if your hand is relaxed. Keep your right hand either palm facing up by the side of your hip or rest it on your abdomen or ribs, as you prefer.
- Inhale through your left nostril while placing pressure on

the right nostril with your ring finger, to block it off very gently.

◆ Breathe in to the top of your inhale without straining, and then pause for a moment before exhaling.

◆ Aim to keep the inhale and exhale of roughly the same duration (you can add the lengthened-exhalation as described below later, if you wish).

◆ Keep breathing in and out of the left nostril for between 1 and 5 minutes.

◆ If your arm gets tired, you can rest it and return to the practice when ready.

◆ Return to natural breathing for a few rounds of breath.

LENGTHENED EXHALE BREATH
AND BREATH COUNTING TOOLS

For a cooling and soothing version of the Basic Yoga (ujjayii) Breath (page 92), lengthen your out-breath, and keep your breath *slow and low*. This means directing attention into – and feeling as though you are 'filling' – the area of your back *below* your shoulders and *above* your low back, where your kidneys sit. Breathing in this way, keeping the tone in your throat subtle and gentle, allows you to breathe both more softly and more fully, and your body and mind will begin to relax deeply.

Follow these instructions to refine ujjayii breath for sleep – focusing down and back with the breath.

◆ Find a pace and timing that is easy and stress-free for you. If you gasp for breath or feel tightness, it's too intense and better to back off.

◆ Fill with breath gently from the bottom to the top (like you'd fill a glass of water). This keeps you from focusing on the upper front third of the lungs, which tends to be more stimulating.

◆ Repeat this breath several times, refining and calming the breath, keeping your face, throat and jaw relaxed. When you're done, return to natural breath, noticing the difference in your body and your mental state.

◆ If you can breathe easily in this way, you may want to add a breath count – for example, start with inhaling for a count of three and exhaling for a count of four. If that's comfortable, you can add a one-beat pause after your exhale. If you start to feel strain, then stop and return to natural breath. Over time and with practice, if your lungs and circulatory system are healthy, you'll be able to extend your exhalation to twice the duration of your inhale and you may find a peaceful natural pause comes in after the outbreath.

PRE-SLEEP BREATHING:
THE 4:7:8 BREATH

If you have healthy lungs or have been practising breathwork, swimming or diving, you may be able to practise breathing in a pattern of a four-count inhale, seven-count retention, and eight-count exhale, popularised by the American integrative medicine guru Dr Andrew Weil. I have used it myself, to help me drop off to sleep after doing some pre-bed yoga, and have seen it work well for others. If you've never done any breathing practices before, it may be too challenging to manipulate your breath like this for long, so if it feels comfortable, you can try one or two rounds, work up to four rounds or more, and then use as desired.

Energising breath practices

Now that we've looked at soothing breath practices, we turn to energising breath practices – and include perfect practices for first thing in the morning, or to use as a mid-afternoon-slump pick-me-up instead of coffee and cake.

Following the instructions for the Basic Yoga Breath (ujjayii), you can energise by making your inhale longer than your exhale.

ENERGISING (SOLAR) RIGHT
NOSTRIL BREATHING (SURYA BHEDANA)

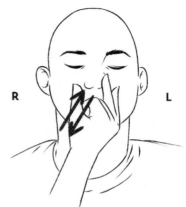

Follow the instructions for Left Nostril Breathing (page 100), but instead inhale and exhale through the right nostril, while gently blocking the left nostril.

If you prefer, you can do this sitting upright as it's more energising.

Start by breathing in and out for the same duration, or practise with a slightly lengthened inhalation throughout the practice for a more stimulating effect.

STRONG, INVIGORATING BREATH:
BREATH OF JOY

This breath is very invigorating, energising and stimulating, and doing it feels slightly playful. The rapid movement of your arms and in-breath stretches the intercostal muscles in your ribcage, activating the rapid-acting stretch receptors in your lungs. According to Amy Weintraub, a leading expert on yoga for depression, this breath has anti-depressive and mood-lifting qualities. The first inhalation (arms forward) makes you breathe into your diaphragm. The second inhalation (arms to the side) gets you breathing into your upper back. The third inhalation (arms up) encourages you to breathe into your upper chest, up by your collarbones. Adding the forward bend on the exhale stretches the long muscles that line the spine, and putting your head down below your heart is refreshing and energising, bringing blood flow into your face and head.

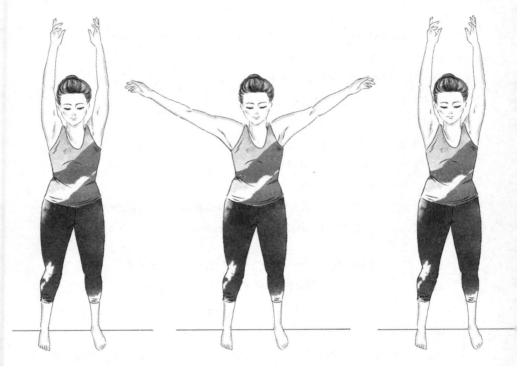

- Stand with your feet wider than hip-distance apart. Keep your knees bent gently, and to make it a bit more lively you can bounce up on to the balls of your feet on the in-breaths, keeping your knees slightly bent.
- Take three sharp 'sips' of breath in through your nose. Each 'sip' has a corresponding arm movement. You'll bend forwards as you exhale. Use the more activating strong ujjayii breath for these.
- Sip 1. Inhale through the nose and gently swing your arms up in front of you, parallel to the floor.
- Sip 2. Inhale through the nose again, swinging your arms open to the sides in a T shape, opening your chest.
- Sip 3. Inhale and lift your arms up above your head.

◆ Exhale. Exhale through your nose sharply while lowering your arms to rest on your thighs as you bend forwards gently. Before the exhale, you may choose to add a 'ha' sound. This means you will exhale through your mouth. I 'brace' the exhale, adding a slight brake to the forward bend instead of sending the arms through the centre of the legs. This helps to make the forward bend safer for anyone with back injuries, adds a grounding quality and minimises lightheadedness.

The arm movements are: front, side, up, down. The breath movement is: in, in, in, out.

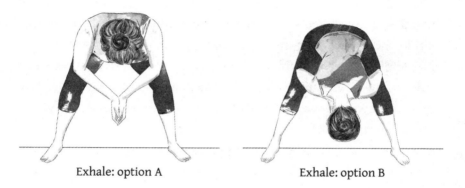

Exhale: option A   Exhale: option B

When you shouldn't do Breath of Joy

You should avoid this practice if you have untreated high blood pressure, acute anxiety, a head injury, migraines or glaucoma. If you have limited movement in your arms or find the breathing overstimulating, you can make smaller movements with your arms, keeping your upper arms closer to your sides. If you have low blood pressure, do this exercise at a slower pace and bend forward on your exhale more slowly.

Parents, mom-somnia, breathing the baby down

When I teach yoga for sleep courses to mixed groups, there is always at least one mother who says that she slept well her entire life until she had her baby. It is often, but not always, the first baby that seems to 'break' her sleep. Parents of newborns need to be hyper-vigilant because human babies are defenceless to a greater extent than most other mammals. Parents' sleep patterns start mirroring babies' sleep patterns so that they can take care of them, but this leaves them exhausted. While adults sleep in five to seven sleep cycles of between 60 and 90 minutes each, moving first from non-rapid-eye movement (NREM, body-restoring sleep) to REM (brain active) sleep, this is completely different to infants' sleep cycles. Babies have short sleep cycles of 10–40 minutes, and fall immediately into REM sleep. Any new parent will tell you that babies also wake to feed frequently.

The new parent often adopts infant sleep patterns and can hold on to them long after the little one has outgrown them. While I suspect this may have been the case for some people in every generation of parents, I also suspect that it has got worse.

It's particularly important for parents to get some nervous system repair because babies, before they can speak and understand language, respond to the physical cues in their world: touch, tone of voice, light and dark, warmth and cold. A baby's cry is designed to alarm us so we will respond to their needs for food and safety, and for often stressed and anxious new parents it's a big challenge to convey a calm and soothing state to a baby who is tense and shrieking. Also, since infants sleep up to two-thirds of the day but in a very different pattern to the adult's consolidated night-time sleep, if new parents don't have enough sleep to drop into the latter stages of REM-heavy sleep this can cause mental weariness and exacerbate post-partum depression.

If you're a new parent you can use the practices in this step to help you through the sleepless nights and to soothe your tired nerves. To get into the 'rest and digest' state with your baby, do breathing practices with babe-in-arms. If you learn the Basic Yoga (ujjayii) Breath (page 92), lengthened exhale breath (page 101) and three-part breathing (page 97), you can do these while nursing or feeding your baby, or to calm your own body before holding your little one.

Restorative postures bolster a tired body, as they provide feelings of support. Meditation, as found in Step 3, can help with replenishing the mental resilience lost when sleep is sparse.

NEW PARENTS' RESCUE KIT

* Learn soothing breaths not only to help settle your baby, but to calm yourself as well!
* Approach and hold a crying baby with deep breaths, slowing down your own heart rate.
* Do some simple stretches throughout the day so your body doesn't hold on to tension unnecessarily.
* Repair your ability to really rest by doing restorative poses when your baby is taking a nap – these can be as restful, or even more so, than brief naps. One favourite is the Diamond Pose on page 119. It feels totally supportive – it's great for a new parent to feel propped up and held. The chest opening in the pose is great for counteracting the effects of curling your arms forwards to hold and feed an infant.
* A 20-minute meditation session, according to research into Transcendental Meditation, can be ten times more restful than sleep to your tired mental state. See page 142 for more on this.
* Sing soothing songs or hum to your baby – this soothes both of you. The bedtime lullaby has some neuroscience to back it up – singing involves a long exhale, which calms your nervous system, and the sound you make tones the vagus nerve, which is a key to soothing and calming your body and brain.

Kids + Teens: under pressure

It seems there is tremendous academic pressure on many kids now. I know that in my own younger years I had few tools for dealing with pressure. It took a huge toll on my sleep, and I know the student years embedded some of my worst sleep habits.

I studied for a degree away from home, and like most of my fellow students, I kept irregular sleep hours: doing all-nighters before exams or papers were due, almost always going to sleep late, sleeping in and becoming constitutionally incapable of sleeping during the night. Most of the people I was with broke our sleep habits during this time.

Julia lived in my dorm. She was the exception when it came to managing student stress, and got through the notoriously difficult pre-med programme at our university much more easily than any of her classmates. She never seemed stressed as she steadily slayed term papers and aced exams. She would quietly disappear into her room, and when asked what she was doing, she'd offer one word: 'Yoga'. She'd learned stretches, breathing practices and meditation in childhood when her parents spent time in a yoga community, and she grew up using yoga's tools as second nature.

It wasn't until after my student days that I discovered yoga, and always sort of wished that I could do it all over, knowing what Julia knew. When Paul, one of my yoga students, approached me after class one day to ask if one of my 'yoga for insomnia' workshops would work for his pre-teen daughter, Anna, I was happy to work with her. Paul said Anna had always slept well, but now had difficulty getting up in the morning and was really groggy all day, struggling under the weight of exams, and he was worried she was up all night.

If Anna learned now how to manage stress and regulate her nervous system when she got tense, these skills might be 'normal' for her to rely on later, and she'd likely avoid the full-blown insomnia, academic panic or depression many kids her age experience. She might even find exams less stressful if she could bring in the calming breathing practices that I teach in Sleep Recovery. If Anna acquired these tools before her teen years set in, my hope was she'd get through her schooling with a bit more ease and grace.

I arrived at Paul's house and he disappeared upstairs to find Anna. I noticed her tired-looking eyes, her long, bony limbs, and that she was rounding her shoulders forward like pre-teen girls do. When her dad introduced us, she nodded at me and kid-mumbled a pleased-to-meet-you. We rolled out three mats and settled on the floor, sitting on sofa cushions.

I guided Anna and her dad through the Simple Sleep Sequence. Anna followed along with the stretches, and after a few, she began rocking back and forth and wiggling her toes playfully. She became noticeably calmer, and her little limbs seemed heavier. She was still awake enough for me to review the poses with her. I showed them to her on the 'cheat sheet' sequence I had printed off and brought with me. I asked her if she liked doing the exercises – she nodded yes – and we brainstormed how she could move some things around in her room to give her space to do poses after reading, before lights-out at night.

During the poses, I was checking Anna's breathing: it started out short and jagged, fighting against her rounded-forward shoulders. Anna was loose-limbed and flexible, so the poses settled her body easily, but her breathing was still relatively shallow and jagged.

We went back over the Basic Yoga Breath (page 44) and I taught her to lengthen her exhale (page 101), so that her heartbeat slowed down. Next, I taught her the three-part breathing (page 97). We moved through each of the three parts, and she was asleep before we reached the last part, which moves the breath up and down the body in a wave. Paul and I decided to let her rest a bit, and exited the living room quietly.

That was the last time I saw Anna, but I heard from Paul the following week:

We did the yoga routine together for a week after your session. This week she wanted to try it on her own with the drawings you gave her. She's been falling asleep with the sequence and breath practices sheet next to the bed. She looks so much more relaxed, and I notice she is doing the breathing without my having to remind her.

It's great when parents can join their children in doing Sleep Recovery yoga: it never hurts to have those tools and skills to hand, to help remind and support them when needed. It's not unusual to see a much stronger effect in fewer sessions for young people: while adults can see real progress in long-term insomnia after the first session, they often take four to six sessions to really shift their patterns because their breathing, nervous system and body tension are so entrenched.

Starting young with sustainable tools for healthy sleep can make a deep imprint and, as was the case with Anna, one session can make a massive difference. If they practise what they're given, simple lessons can make a lasting impression on young people.

PART 2:
REPAIR YOUR
RELAXATION RESPONSE

There is a little crimson book from the 1970s that holds a simple secret. In it, Harvard Medical School researcher Herbert Benson and author Miriam Klipper describe the phenomenon they refer to in the book's title, *The Relaxation Response*: a physical *state of deep rest* in which our heart rate slows down, the rates of inhale and exhale slow down, blood flow returns to our limbs and circulation improves. As you slip into this state, you may find yourself yawning – a sign that your body is releasing tension. You might hear your stomach gurgle, as the digestive wave called peristalsis kicks back in. Things start to change from the locked-down feelings that accompany mild to intense stress to a sense of greater fluidity and ease.

This relaxed state is *anabolic*, which means that in terms of our metabolism, it builds us back up. Most of us know the word anabolic from the term 'anabolic steroids' – the stuff weightlifters use to build muscles artificially. Being in the relaxation response doesn't puff up our bodies in an unhealthy way, but instead builds us back up organically and naturally.

On the other end of the metabolic spectrum, stress is *catabolic*, which means that it breaks down molecules to get the energy out of them. When we're stressed, our bodies get ready to burn energy quickly – to run away or fight. But since we're stressed too often and our lives can be sedentary, our bodies are mobilising energy we don't need and can't use, so if we're stressed, we can use up our reserves, end up depleted, and develop stress-related conditions such as adrenal fatigue, anxiety, chronic fatigue syndrome or depression, which can relate to overusing the stress hormone cortisol. Our growing inability to get to sleep, stay asleep or find sleep refreshing is part of the same phenomenon.

On the other hand, getting into the relaxation response, and allowing our bodies to rest and digest, helps us to counter the effects of stress *immediately* – and those effects build over time.

Sleep research shows that the 'sleep debt' we rack up, either by sleeping too little, staying up too late or through inability to get to sleep, can't be repaid like paying back money owed. The body just does its best to even out over time, and if we learn to give in to our tiredness and put rest back into our lives we *can* re-resource ourselves. The deep rest we experience in the relaxation response is not exactly the same as sleep, but can actually be maintained for longer, because we can consciously decide to spend time there, throughout the day, putting energy back on the grid when we need it.

Reconnecting to the relaxation response can stop us from loading up on stimulants, and can recondition our capacity to get to sleep, stay asleep and sleep more deeply, and help us feel both calm and alert during the day. The restorative postures in this step support your body and help your nervous system to rest and enter the relaxation response. I found these practices incredibly valuable at a time when doing more active practices wasn't possible.

Restorative practices: put energy back on the grid

One summer, I was stuck at home following a painful operation on both of my feet. I was struggling with post-operative insomnia and I wasn't able to practise yoga as usual. While the surgery would end near-constant foot pain I'd had for several years, in the short term the wounds were agonising and immobilising. I couldn't walk, cycle or swim until the skin and bones healed. Not moving around left me tense, wired and fizzing with unspent energy. This was a disaster for my sleep: I needed to find a solution that helped me calm the anxieties that come up with intense physical pain and help me get my circulation going without depleting me. A friend gave me Judith Lasater's book *Relax and Renew* for my birthday, which took place soon after the operation. In Lasater's book I learned how to do yoga poses that didn't require me to stand up, and soothed my body profoundly while easing out the tension that had built up. I've since learned how to use pared-back and easy restoratives to energise myself after a messy night's sleep or to restore my energy in the middle of a busy afternoon. The instructions are here, and you can see how they helped two exhausted parents, Beth and Nicole, after the instructions that follow.

RESTORATIVE POSES BUILD
THE RELAXATION RESPONSE

Doing one or more of these restorative postures can help you face your day with more resilience. You can do a single posture for up to 15 minutes, or do three over the course of between 20 and 45 minutes. A simple restorative session promotes calm, perspective, and better, more sustainable energy. Doing these poses in the morning is like 'mopping up after a bad night's sleep'. In the morning or afternoon, these poses don't interfere with your body's appetite for sleep (often called the *sleep drive*) but they do keep us from walking around in a frazzled yet depleted state, so you avoid falling into the trap of getting false energy from caffeine or stress hormones.

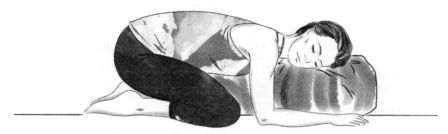

Extended Child's Pose

This pose is like curling up in the foetal position. You rest the front of your body from your forehead down to your chest and abdomen on two or more firm bed pillows or a long firm sausage-shaped cushion called a bolster, like the ones sometimes found on the arms of a sofa. The body is curled forward, with the front of the legs and lower back stretching, but the abdomen is protected and supported. I like to imagine that all the stress, tension and worry in my body are like a thick blue-black inky substance and that when I exhale, the cushions absorb the inky sludge like an old-fashioned ink blotter, or like soft porous earth absorbs rainwater.

This pose is natural to children, as it recalls being in the womb, and it's not unusual to find a little one comforting himself in this position. With your forehead down, your attention goes inward, allowing you to feel very protected and safe. The posture gently draws circulation into the abdomen and lungs as the blood flow moves downwards with gravity. It can feel like a tremendous relief during or at the end of a depleting day to come to this position, which can feel like it's protecting us from the world: it's a sense of elemental 'coming home'.

You will need a bolster or two, or three firm bed pillows and a rolled-up blanket (optional) and a rolled-up towel (optional).

- Come on to your hands and knees in a box position.
- Place your big toes together and move your knees apart wider than your hips, and bring your bottom down towards your heels. If this is too difficult, you can place a rolled-up blanket beneath your bottom, and if your feet or ankles are tight you can place a rolled-up towel under the front of your ankles.
- Fold forward and rest your abdomen, chest and forehead on the bolster or pillows.
- As you fold on to your supporting cushions, stack your hands one on top of the other, and rest your forehead on the top hand.
- Breathe consciously and slowly. With the breath, a simple visualisation helps to focus the mind and to amplify the effect of this passive, supported stretch.

You can use this image: The mercury in an old-fashioned thermometer rises and falls slowly. When you start to inhale, imagine your breath like the mercury rising, filling up from the tip of your tailbone, and as you breathe, trace up the back of your body from the low back through the shoulders to curl up over the back of your skull, coming to the crown of your head at the end of the in-breath. You slow down and even out your inhalation by visualising it moving up the back of your body. As you breathe out, imagine your breath washing down the front of your body, from the forehead down, smoothing out your face and jaw, softening your throat, stomach and lower abdomen as you exhale.

- ◆ Do this for at least 10 breaths. If you're comfortable there, you may find you drop into a deep relaxation or a mini-snooze.
- ◆ Remember to turn your head to one side first and then to the other, so your neck stretches out evenly on both sides.

Feet Up and Rest

I love that this pose is both remarkably simple and rather dramatic in its effect. The trick is in getting the angles right. If you lie down on the floor and put your feet on the seat of a chair or a sofa, you can rest the back of your calves there. If the height works well, you can stack your kneecaps over your hips.

This angle gives you one of the three important actions of the position: opening up your belly and chest by releasing the iliopsoas muscle. Starting inside the upper inner thigh is a very deep, very important protection muscle called the psoas muscle (pronounced so-as), which travels over the front of your pelvis, where it meets the iliacus muscle, so named because it travels over the protruding front-

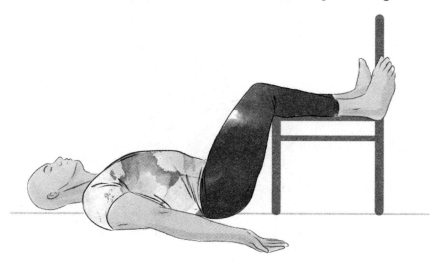

of-hip bone called the ilium. The psoas then fans out from the lower spine to attach at the mid-back (the 12th vertebra of the thoracic spine). When we are tense, fearful or protective, this muscle tightens us up into a protective stance, like a boxer hunches forwards. This tightens the diaphragm, making it harder to breathe. It happens naturally – we round forward to protect the vital inner organs that are left exposed because our ribs only go so far down. In 'Feet Up and Rest' pose, the top of your long thigh bone drops down and back into your pelvic socket and relaxes the tension in the psoas muscle.

The second action of this pose is that it is an *inversion* (meaning upside down). Inversions help to drain fluid out of the legs and feet, promoting the flow of lymph, which has the important function in the immune system of carrying infection-fighting white blood cells around the body.

The third action of the pose is that it places a little extra pressure on the heart and lungs, and fills them with blood flow. It may also be the case that the heart and lungs press on the aorta, one of the main

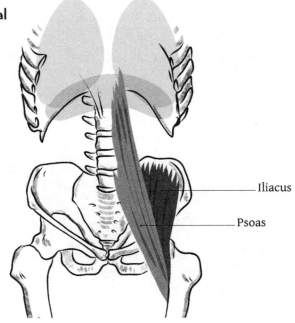

Some internal postural muscles

Iliacus

Psoas

Posture tip

Move your bottom away from the legs of the chair or sofa so you maintain a gentle curve in your lower back. Make sure the place where your legs meet your torso is soft and relaxed. The front of your pelvis (pubic bone) will drop down when you're in the right spot. When this happens, your legs will relax, the front of your hips and thighs will release, the tops of your thigh bones will nestle into the back of the pelvis, and this will relax the lower back. Adjust until this feels comfortable.

valves in the heart, which sits to the back, and this pressure may slow down the heart rate.

As for the posture, the version where you place your calves on the seat of a chair is my favourite for the middle of the day. In between therapy clients, I will often take five minutes in this position with my legs up, and my head will clear as I breathe deeply at first, and then more shallowly as I start to relax properly.

This pose can be done at the end of an active day to rejuvenate, or after a long flight to restore circulation to the feet and legs. However, legs-up poses aren't good for those who are menstruating, or for heavily pregnant women or people with gastric reflux or heart disease or restricted breathing conditions.

You'll need a chair with a stable (non-rolling) base for the chair version, or a sofa with its seat low enough so that you can rest your calves on it comfortably, and a rolled-up towel or blanket or a cushion (optional).

+ Lie on your back in front of the chair or sofa.
+ Keep your back on the floor, and swing your calves on to the sofa cushions or seat of the chair.
+ Place a rolled-up towel or blanket under the curve of your neck or use a low cushion to support your head if needed.

• Find the natural curve in your lower back, so that your back is not flattened into the floor as if in an abdominal crunch, nor is your low back dramatically arched into a chest-thrust-forward position. A gentle curve in the lower back is enough, with the sacrum resting evenly on the floor and your shoulders and the back of your skull also resting evenly on the floor.

• If your shins roll out, this can compress your lower back. To prevent this happening, tuck in your shins and hold them in place at hip-width apart using a blanket, or loop a yoga belt loosely around your shins and tighten it until your shins are hip-width apart.

• Stay here with your arms open out to the sides and palms facing upwards, or gently rest your hands, palms down, on your abdomen if that feels safer or more comfortable.

• You may find you are more comfortable if your chin is slightly lower than your forehead, so that the back of your neck is naturally curved but not flattened down into the floor. This lets your face and neck muscles relax and release their grip.

Legs Up the Wall Variation

The above practice can also be done with your legs straight and your heels resting on a wall. It's important to be close enough to the wall for your legs to be supported but to keep your bottom far enough away that there's no tension in your hips and hamstrings.

For this, I often place a firm cushion under the sacrum/lower back. Also, a belt looped firmly around the shins (or a blanket draped over your feet and tucked into the wall) can be especially helpful when your legs and hip flexors begin to relax, which can make your legs drop out to the sides unevenly and create tension in the lower back and groin. If your body is trying to keep your legs UP when it's tired, it's going to expend unnecessary energy when the point of doing the poses is to feel more rested. The belt holds everything in place and allows your hip flexors to relax, because they don't have to stabilise your legs.

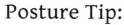

Posture Tip:

M aintain the gentle arch in the lower back, and relax at the hip flexor crease. If the pubic bone is higher than the front pelvic bones, the pose will be less relaxing and breathing will be more inhibited, as the forward tilt in the pelvis can make the diaphragm in the middle ribcage area contract and tighten.

The Deluxe Rest Pose (Diamond Pose)

This resting position takes a bit of set-up because it supports your body in very specific places so that where it's been holding tension it can relax very deeply. It brings circulation and blood flow into the lower abdomen – the base of the body, the digestive and reproductive organs. It also opens up your chest and your head rests back, taking the weight and pressure off your neck.

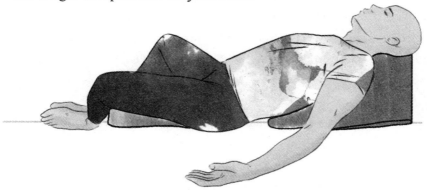

I particularly like this one as a mid-afternoon rest during the slump time. It gives me a chance to replenish and leaves me feeling more awake and nurtured. Its standard yoga name is supta baddha konasana (supine bound angle pose) but is often called 'goddess pose'. To make it more gender-neutral and memorable, I call it Diamond Pose or The Deluxe Rest Pose.

When the pose is set up, you will be seated with your bottom propped up a bit, your back resting on an inclined cushion so that your chest opens up, and your head supported so that it rests back, releasing tension in your face and neck. Your legs will open out butterfly-style, knees pointing to either side. Resting your outer thighs on cushions or blocks will support the opening out of your hips.

You will need a bolster and something stable to prop it on to make a slant, or two large, firm cushions. The ones from the seat or back of the sofa work well. Unfortunately, this doesn't work with a futon sofa!

You will also need two simple yoga blocks, which are shaped like bricks, to provide support under your thighs in order to release the grip of your hip flexors and protect your knees. Alternatively, you can use two piles of thick books that stack up to the same size – between 7 and 12cm (3–5in) high – or two firm, evenly sized throw pillows if they are at least 7cm (3in) high – or use two on each side, making sure the sides are even. Yoga blocks aren't expensive, however, and will save you the hassle of relocating the contents of your living room. You may also need a folded blanket or smaller cushion for your bottom, a cushion or rolled up towel for your neck, and some sort of padding for your forearms. Make sure you have your yoga blocks and additional padding where you can easily reach them once you are in the pose.

- Cross your bolsters or cushions into a T-shape, so that you have a slant – a 45-degree incline.
- An option is to place a smaller cushion, folded blanket or flat block at the lower, shorter end of the bolster. This is for you to

sit on, and prevent a really dramatic curve in the lower back – some people find this starts pinching.

+ Sit at the lower end of the bolster and lie back along the bolster's length, with your head supported by the top of the bolster.

+ You can put a cushion or rolled-up towel behind your neck to support it, but don't rest your head on something too high or this will push your head forward. If you spend much of your day looking at a screen, driving or carrying heavy things, it will feel good to let your head rest back, lengthen the front of your throat and let the back of your neck release.

+ Make sure your chin doesn't tilt upwards – if this happens, you'll be looking up towards the ceiling and your face, neck and eyes won't relax completely. Instead, your forehead should be a little higher than your chin.

+ Now, bend your knees so they point outwards into a butterfly position, with the insides of your thighs to the ceiling and the soles of your feet touching. Move your feet as far away as possible while they still touch. This minimises the strain on your knees, opens up your hips and creates a more relaxed position.

+ Put cushions or blocks under your outer thighs to support them, making sure the height is exactly even on both sides. If the cushions or blocks are too low, your hips will stay tight. If you let your thighs rest on enough height and they are supported, your hips will open effortlessly.

+ A final option is to rest folded blankets, blocks, firm cushions or books under your forearms, as though you were sitting in an armchair. This allows your arms to release their tension, and takes pressure off your shoulder joints.

+ Stay in this position for up to 20 minutes.

+ If it is difficult to relax here initially, try three-part breathing (page 97) to help you release into the posture.

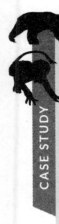

TWO BUSY PARENTS LEARN TO RELAX

Beth and **Nicole** showed up on a Tuesday at 9.30 a.m., each having dropped their 10-year-old boys, both of whom have severe autism, at school. They appear with similarly harried expressions, bundled into puffy overcoats, and hair strewn about by the wintery London rain that seems to come in sideways.

Beth, with thick dark hair, round freckled cheeks and big brown eyes with a thick fringe of lashes, doesn't think of herself as having insomnia but she never really feels *rested*. Each night, she falls into a deep sleep on the sofa in front of the TV with her husband, during their only quiet time together. Between midnight and 1 a.m. they shuffle up to bed. Though Beth, more of a Bear type, has little trouble falling asleep, she wakes each day unrefreshed, with deep black circles under her eyes.

Nicole, more of a Monkey type, is more angular: hair razored to a chin-length bob and piercing eyes, shoulders bunched up around her ears: her constant neck pain and difficulty settling to sleep are not surprising. Nicole sleeps fitfully when she is finally able, and grinds her teeth in the night. As a single parent, she seems to sleep with one eye open: her son often shuffles into her room fresh from one of his frequent nightmares. Though Beth and Nicole's sleep problems are different, they seem to stem from the same root: they have been more or less in new-parent vigilance mode for a decade, and their exhaustion ripples off them.

I roll out the yoga mats in the room. I offer some active yoga moves that they might find familiar. They find it hard to hold the postures, since they are both exhausted. They don't need a workout: they need support.

Their hour with me offers a relatively responsibility-free bubble, but they are still always on call. More so than other parents –

because their children have special needs, they are in constant contact with the school, always ready to respond to emergency calls.

At the end of their first session, I show them the Diamond Pose (page 119).

They watch me assemble all the props with some scepticism, but when I climb into pose they see what effect it has. My body looks relaxed, open, settled: they are sold.

On the first attempt, Nicole fidgets a bit, but Beth is snoring within about 45 seconds. After four minutes or so, even Nicole drops in, her bony body finally draping over the cushions for the last minute as if the stitches that hold her together have loosened. I feel loath to disturb them, but our time is up.

They are surprised at how much looser their legs, shoulders and hips feel, and I notice that a bit of the edge has gone from their faces, at least until they look at their phones. The harried looks return, and I know that the re-patterning of their stress response will be a longer-term project, but a worthwhile one.

I worked with Nicole and Beth for more than a year, doing active yoga postures for 15 minutes of each session to help them transition from hyped-up into a more restful state. We would then go into restorative poses, sometimes three or four of them held for between 5 and 15 minutes each. I added in the breath meditation found in Step 3 (see page 139) in this book about six months in: both women now have tools they can use in a variety of settings.

We kept up our sessions until Beth and her family moved out of London; she had enough energy to start writing the book she'd been putting on hold for years. Nicole went back to work part time in marketing, using her restorative postures between work and picking up her son to give her the energy she needs as a single parent going back to work.

STEP 3

Reclaim
your mind

THE PURPOSE OF THIS STEP is to help you settle and release the grip of your mind so you can sleep better. It's not to help you switch your mind off, but to work *with* it and put it in its right perspective among all the other layers of who and what you are. This will help you to sleep because you will become more capable of 'mental digestion' and you will learn how to shift into the mental states that relate to different conditions in your brain, from waking through to deep sleep.

Of course you can't switch off your mind like a machine. Click: on, click: off. We definitely don't work like that. It's like trying not to think of something: as soon as you try, your lovely creative and rebellious mind will think of exactly that thing! You know what they say: 'Don't think of a pink elephant.' And there it is. A pink elephant right there in your mind. It's also said that 'what you resist will persist', because whatever thought it is, putting up a wall against it bricks it in stronger. Trying not to think about something, or trying to make it go away, keeps it there in negative. Sad, but true.

If you haven't had enough time to deal with the concerns that have piled up throughout the day, it's unsurprising that you will have a parade of thoughts at night when you get into bed and try to quieten your mind. Taking time in your day to *manage the mental inbox* or *clear your plate* is a great way to help you shift into personal care time before bed. If you have a way to lay daily concerns to rest there will be more time for reflection, and your life might start to feel more manageable.

Instead of trying to switch off, it's perhaps more realistic to consider that our thoughts are there for a reason – mostly because the mind is so good at making plans to keep us safe, to see what can be learned from a situation, to apply what we learned in a similar situation to the one we are experiencing now, even if that's not actually helpful.

This is probably part of what makes you great in your own way, but as we have seen, your strengths, when distorted, can also be the things that cause you to go out of balance and lose sleep. What kind of thoughts do you have when you are turning things over in your mind instead of dropping off to sleep?

Here's what it was like for me: for the first part of my adult life, I would lie in my bed at night and my thoughts would be a tangle of fast-moving messages all getting crossed, redirected and ricocheting off one another. They all moved in the direction of catastrophe. Every message was trying to communicate something, but the wires always seemed crossed.

I remember seeing in a movie what old-fashioned telephone switchboards looked like. Someone would call and the operator would pick up the line and have to put the wire into a slot to connect the call. In my head, it was like all the calls would flood in at once, and the connections would cross over, making a lattice of wires unable to be unwoven from one another. The switchboard would go into overload and I, as the operator, the one placing the calls and the one receiving them, would go into meltdown.

Too frequently, we try to put mind over matter, but effective Sleep Recovery recognises that your mind and the *matter* of your body are partners in a delicate dance. If you have begun to calm your body, restoring your ability to rest and digest, you are bound to feel the effects in terms of a more balanced mind. However, there will always be times when your mind is preoccupied – it seems the modern condition is one of having too much to think about and too much to do. Step 3 of Sleep Recovery gives you the principles and practices you need to manage your mind. You'll learn how to use journaling exercises to declutter your mind, discover easy ways to come to your senses, and practise some simple, non-scary meditations to help you manage, clear and sleep-prepare your mind.

Mental patterns and your constitution

When I suffered from insomnia, I had a cluttered, exhausted mind and didn't really understand how to declutter it. Depending on your mental constitution, you might experience a particular kind of repetitive thought before bed.

Monkey type: If you have a creative and flexible mind, when you're out of balance you might be prone to fear and anxiety, dreaming up scenarios of doom and gloom, having slightly paranoid thoughts or conjuring catastrophes.

Tiger type: If your mind is capable of great understanding and intelligence, when you go out of balance you might be consumed with angry, jealous or competitive thoughts, worrying about who has slighted you, comparing or evaluating things during your day, judging and finding yourself or others lacking.

Bear type: If in general you have loving, calm or compassionate thoughts, when you go out of balance you might worry about losing things, feeling overly attached, wanting more (in a greedy way), being concerned about not having enough, or feeling envious that others have more than you.

If you look at both the *content* and the *tone* of your thoughts, you might start to get greater insight into who you are – and how you think – so that you begin to get 'underneath' your thoughts instead of following each one of them as though they were gods. In working with your mind, the idea is not to club it into submission or get it to be the *kind of mind* that it isn't, but what is helpful is to use it as a tool, to allow it to have time to digest things, and then allow it to *rest* after having done its job.

When your thoughts come thick and fast in a torrent, or come parading past clanging cymbals and banging drums, you need to get them to *slow down* and you need to listen to them. Most of us are inundated with information, images and connections all day. We need to deal with the mental inbox. I often think of it like digestion. If you eat a big meal and then exercise directly afterwards, it's hard to digest the meal. You need to spend some time in a relaxed state, to give some space for your food to be broken down. When we don't have any mental downtime, all the information, images and impressions sit with us and we get a case of 'mental indigestion'. Much like physical indigestion causes a reflux or a feeling of food 'repeating'. We can view repetitive thoughts as undigested, or even as indigestible.

One of the things I have experienced, and that rings true for a lot of my clients, is that working through difficult situations can totally take your mind hostage instead of letting it rest and get to sleep. It's natural – you want resolution and it's when you start to get quiet, either before bed or in the middle of the night, that the difficulties of the day really settle in and needle at you. In order to get to sleep, some of us need to 'find a place to put it', whatever the thought or situation might be, so that we can rest and let our unconscious processing do some work on it, too.

You've heard the expression 'Let me sleep on it'? This doesn't mean: let me think about it incessantly, turn it over in my mind, and stay awake all night pondering it. It means: Let me set it aside and see what happens when I get a little distance, and come back to it with a fresh mind and eyes in the morning.

In order to do that, sometimes we need to find a container in which to *put it*. And if you're stuck in one of these positions, with a lot of emotion behind it, it can be hard to 'put it down'. If you experience your sleeplessness as repetitive thoughts 'on a loop' or inability to switch off your mind, and you don't *feel* it as much as *think* it, do the exercises in this step first. However, if your experience is more emotional in nature, Step 4 may be even more useful to you.

Here's what I find useful, and have seen work with my clients. When we put our bodies into bed at the end of a long, busy day, it can be the only time we've stopped and had a chance to process the day at all. Any thoughts, worries, resentments, concerns or slights can arise very naturally and cause anxiety, worry or simple preoccupation. They've been waiting all day for attention. I call this the thought parade, because it can be so noisy and busy!

When you can't sleep and the thoughts come marching in, I suggest you slow down your thoughts by writing them down, let them play out, and look *underneath* them to identify the emotion that's generating them. The physical act of writing – the material sensory touch and movement of hand, pen or pencil and paper – brings our thoughts together and can help us find resolution.

Start with the basics. Find a pen or pencil and a piece of paper or notebook. If you absolutely must use a screen, go ahead, but it's far better to do this by hand. If you hate writing, try recording a voice note. The act of speaking and listening to it afterwards may also help you to reflect and get it off your chest.

- Write down every crazy thought you have. This alone can be helpful.
- Let all the different conflicting thoughts out: 'On the one hand...' and 'On the other hand...' If there is conflict within you, and you have two or more perspectives, write from each one separately to get them all down on paper.
- Play the thoughts and assumptions to the end, asking: and then what?
- Then have a look at them.
- And decide to put your list aside and give yourself some time to think it through or take action during the day or later in the week. And then honour this by sticking to it.

The Captain's Log

Another journaling exercise recalls Captain Jean-Luc Picard from the starship Enterprise (of the *Star Trek* series), who kept a regular 'Captain's Log'. I suggest that clients keep a journal in which they can do a brain-dump, reviewing the day's events and setting aside anything that needs to be noted for tomorrow – without getting into an exhaustive to-do list. If something interpersonal is causing concern, write it down. If something at work is unsettled, write it down. Write thoughts, intuitions and the sense of the situation, and keep writing until you are ready to set it aside. Some people need to feel that no one will find their brain-dump, in which case I suggest tearing it up, or disposing of it before bed or in the morning. Others find keeping a journal to which they can refer later very helpful for resolving the difference between late-night anxieties – which are often disproportionate – and daytime reality.

* Set a timer for between 2 and 5 minutes, and free-write.
* Don't take your pen off the page for the time you've set. Keep writing, even if you are writing 'I don't know what to write' or repeating the same thing over and over.

CHOOSE A WRITING PROMPT

A third way to journal is to put one of the prompts from the list below at the top of a page and do 2 to 5 minutes on only that. You may want to use only one prompt, or you might take 10–25 minutes and burn through several. The prompts are:

* What's really bothering me is:
* What I want to say but can't is:
* The thing I'm most afraid of is:
* About this situation: What can I change? What can't I change?
* If my wisest self were in charge, s/he would:

Here are some prompts for repetitive thoughts, and ways to write through these thoughts:

Repetitive thought	Working it through might look like this:
The worst thing will happen: Catastrophic thoughts.	Get realistic: what is the likelihood that the catastrophe will happen? Put a percentage on it. Make a mini catastrophe plan: if it happens, what might you do? Having 'catastrophe plans' can make for good comedy or can help you feel relieved. Picture a scenario with a neutral or positive outcome. Defuse the negative fantasy by asking, 'Okay, so if that horrible thing happens then something comes next – what is the next thing?'
I need to be in control of this: Controlling thoughts.	Figure out what IS in your control and what isn't. Hint: trying to control other people, places or things usually doesn't work. Recognising what is in your power to change, and what isn't, is a path to greater peace.
I'm right! They're wrong! Persecuting thoughts.	Get a sense of humour: realise that everyone always thinks they're right all the time, and this is clearly possible! Ask: what would the other person need to believe in order to hold their perspective? You can disagree, but understanding enables you to loosen your self-righteousness and calm down.
I got it wrong! Self-critical thoughts.	Develop compassion for yourself: Repeat after me, 'I did my best.' You can write out what you might do differently in a similar situation next time. If you were in the wrong, you might even write out an apology. Nothing helps us to sleep like a clear conscience.

Repetitive thought	Working it through might look like this:
An aggravating or difficult thought keeps coming up: Emotionally-laden thoughts.	Listen to the thought, focus on the FEELING behind it: I'm feeling: sad, angry, resentful etc. Then write out why you don't want to feel that way. Then say to yourself: It's okay.
Worried about losing something or someone: Anxious thoughts.	Ask: How will I put one foot in front of the other, and find one good thing in each day, if I lose this thing, or this person? How can I find something meaningful, even if there is sadness?
I'm worried about losing my health.	Ask: How can I live a good life with the health and time that I do have? What do I value the most? How can I live with that in mind for the time I have?

Cathy, who is retired and has suffered from sleep problems for many years, says, 'I was always exhausted and couldn't seem to think straight all day, but when I'd get into bed at night, my mind would seize upon repetitive thoughts. I couldn't let go of things, I would replay conversations or situations in my head.' When Cathy began to do some journaling before her bedtime yoga routine, she found that her mind was more settled and it was easier to focus on her breathing as she moved. With a more settled mind, the stretches seemed to go deeper. If during her morning wake-up routine, particularly focused on energising movements and breath, she had intrusive thoughts or felt preoccupied, she'd write down the daily to-dos and found that not only was her sleep improving because the morning practices brought stimulation at the right time of day, but it was easier to let go, and to then manage enjoyable daily activities, be more creative with her (many) grandchildren's birthday gifts, feel less preoccupied and more actively 'on top of things'.

Mindfulness: come to your senses

Mindfulness is a term used to describe adaptations of ancient Buddhist practices which have recently become widely recognised for their therapeutic power. It's about being aware – mindful – of the 'here and now' and observing and accepting feelings and thoughts without judgement. Put simply, it's about getting out of your thinking-mind and both observing impassively and coming to your senses – literally – which is often exactly what we need when our thoughts are spiralling out of control. The BELL technique – Breathe, Expand your awareness, Listen, Look – is a mindfulness practice that takes your mind out of the stories you tell yourself and brings you into the five senses and the present moment. It's very, very simple. You don't even need to close your eyes. You can do this practically any time, provided you're in a generally safe environment. Even if there's something emotional happening, you can practise this and start to shift your brain chemistry.

Try these instructions to come back to the present moment, move out of stress and enter a more rested state.

- Breathe simply and easily and see if you can feel your back in your seat or your feet on the ground.
- Now take two or three deep breaths and then expand your awareness: notice what's happening around you.
- Look around the room or out of a window and see what's there. Name three things you can see – start with an object or a colour.
- Shut your eyes, and notice three things you can hear when you listen.
- You may continue the exercise to note three things you can touch, smell or even taste.

Keep it simple and practise it often to come back to present-time mindfulness.

Train your brain to sleep

The electrical activity in your brain, when shown visually on a monitor called an electro-encephalogram (EEG), looks like the waves in a choppy sea, with peaks and troughs, ups and downs spiking up and receding. It allows for new connections.

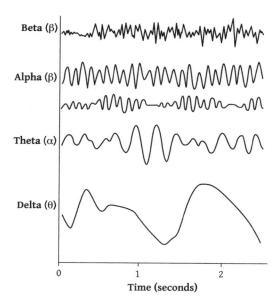

These are the different brainwave patterns, all of which are needed in a healthy functioning brain. The way your brain works habitually relates to how you use your mind and body: not only your thoughts and mental focus but also the cues from your body and breath, as we explored in the previous steps. If you don't sleep well because of an overactive mind, it's a good idea to make sure you don't spend all your time in the beta-wave brain state but cultivate the other states. The yoga, mindfulness, restorative postures and meditation practices are like cross-training for your brain, reconditioning your ability to be in downtime: daydreaming, meditating, or experiencing a sense of wonder or awe.

Beta waves predominate in an awake, active brain. Being able to tackle your to-do list and respond to emails efficiently but then being able to put these down during your break time shows balanced beta-wave activity. Lying in the dark ruminating on the previous day, and feeling anxiety or fear about past or upcoming events, may correspond with overactive beta-wave activity.

Alpha waves are associated with a relaxed waking state, or a transition from waking to sleep. Sitting quietly, simply observing your breath or a pleasant view, listening to music without distraction or watching the kettle boil and feeling your feet on the floor might correspond with balanced alpha.

Theta waves are associated with the sleep state. They may be present when you're awake if you're feeling day-dreamy or trance-like, staring off into space. Entering into a visionary state during meditation, visualisation, spiritual practice or the use of psychedelics could induce theta-wave patterns while we're awake.

Delta waves are found in the deepest sleep state, when you're dreaming. If you're feeling sluggish and brain-fogged in the morning, possibly due to an alarm going off in the middle of a dream, it may be because you've still got a lot of delta-wave activity. You may feel a little trippy and disoriented if you've got a lot of delta activity while awake.

Depending on your disposition and your habits, you may tend towards being overactive or underactive in different brainwave states. People who are highly stressed have a high concentration of beta waves and may struggle to drop into alpha as a precursor for cascading into the sleep states of delta and theta. Practising meditation can help you train your brain to make the transition into sleep more easily – not switching off but 'dropping down'. Meditating regularly helps you to reduce beta waves and sympathetic nervous system activity to move from the alpha- into the delta-wave states of the relaxation-response state more easily. This is a great reason to practise the meditation styles in this step.

Repair your relaxation response

When you sleep, your brain goes through a cycle of different types of activity (see page 133). Sleep Recovery essentially trains your brain (along with every other part of you) to go from active to more relaxed; specifically through meditation, you learn to relax deeply on cue and, with your eyes closed, you enter states that align with the brainwave patterns of sleep and dreaming. This makes it easier to fall asleep and stay asleep, but if you have trouble sleeping at night, meditating during the day restores your energy by giving you a bit of the brain activity you would see during your night's sleep.

The basics of meditation involve very little, and the practice is actually very simple, even if it's not always easy. It is completely free, involves nothing to buy, nothing to prove to anyone, is always accessible literally anywhere, and has incredible benefits for your body, your nervous system, your mind and your sense of happiness – but astonishingly, very few people tap into it.

I can understand this: the first time I tried to sit down and meditate, closing my eyes in a silent room, I nearly imploded. I beat myself up because *in theory,* closing my eyes and sitting still 'should' be easy. The clock was so loud I could hear every single tick, as if it were right up against my ear. Every noise took my mind off into a thousand directions. I kept thinking of *things.* Every. Thing. All of them. Emails needing a reply. Bills unopened on the kitchen table. What to have for dinner. Every itch I ever had came back at the same time, *begging* to be scratched. My feet fell asleep. My back hurt. On and on: you get it.

I came up with every excuse imaginable to not just sit there, because I had never learned to *just sit there.* It was a lot like trying to get to sleep, and the operative word was TRYING. As soon as you stop trying, you stop gripping on to the thoughts and feelings. For me, it feels like saying to myself, 'Oh, okay... that... um-hm. That's okay... and *breathe.*' It's said very *lightly,* with sense of humour. I think I've learned to find my thoughts, itches and twitches amusing, even the intense ones. I can say to myself: 'Wow, that's a pretty catastrophic thought' and internally nod: 'Yep. That's what it is.'

Here's the diagram that I draw for my students.

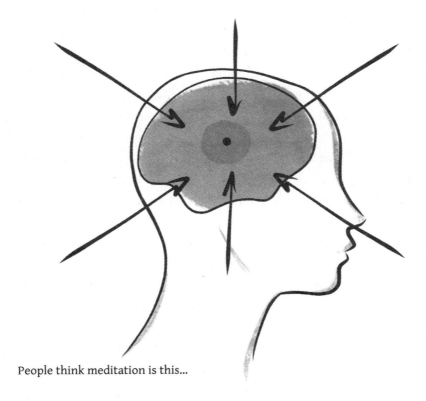

People think meditation is this...

I used to think (mistakenly) that meditating meant I would focus (the straight arrows) on THE THING (the dot) and that my mind, if I was doing it right, would STAY ON THE THING. But it kept going away from the thing. And I kept getting annoyed and frustrated that it wouldn't STAY ON THE THING. Which made my body more tense, and made me more likely to fidget, which made me more annoyed, and took my mind off THE THING. Or I'd focus on the thing, and then the THING WOULD DISAPPEAR and I'd have nothing there, or fall asleep or think SOME OTHER THING. And I'd get annoyed at that.

But here's the thing. Meditation isn't about THE THING. It is a process of giving your mind SOMETHING, a place for your mind to return to because it will definitely wander, because that is what minds do. They have thought after thought until you are dead. And trying not to think will make you crazy. The key is to focus on THE THING and then notice, with amusement, when my mind goes away from it and that it is doing SOME OTHER THING and then say to myself gently: 'Okay, okay... back to the thing.'

This is what meditation is: the process of going from THE thing to other things, and back to THE thing. You go from the focus of the meditation (a mantra, the breath, etc) into thoughts, and then when you notice you've trailed off away from the focus you bring it back kindly. And doing that, guiding the mind back like you'd redirect a wayward toddler away from the side of a swimming pool without freaking her out – is just a gentle redirect, here we go, alley-oop, I'm picking you up and putting you down somewhere else that's better for you.

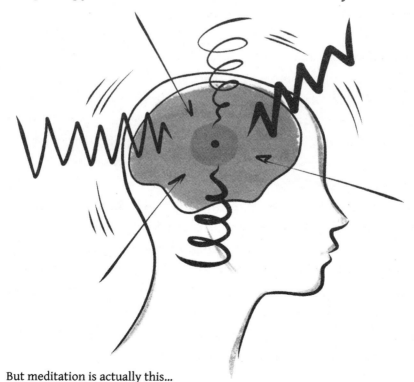

But meditation is actually this...

Our society and its demands have patterned us away from gently directing our minds back to a focus. Meditation isn't actually *doing nothing* but it does involve doing something *very different* to what you may be accustomed to. It's gently asking your mind: 'Can you come back here so you can rest?' When you do it for long enough, all the unprocessed thoughts and emotions that have been sitting beneath the surface come up. In Step 1, I described how yoga stretches offer your body a clean-out: meditation is like a clean-out for your mind. When you sit to meditate, if your mind is very active it feels like you've turned out all the contents of the closet on to the floor and are confronted with it all. My meditation teachers gave me the idea that when my mind is really active in meditation, it's not that I'm doing it wrong: there's just a lot to sort through. In the UK, we get this white chalky sediment on our electric tea kettles that clogs them up. It's a mineral limescale deposit that needs to be removed so the water in the kettle can run clear. Meditation does the mental equivalent of lifting off the limescale deposits. After a while, you get a sense of humour about it: up and out it goes. It's just *stuff*.

At the other extreme, when my mind isn't overactive with all manner of stuff, I can often feel like I'm falling asleep in meditation. I used to think that this was also *doing it wrong*. My meditation teachers gave me a different way of thinking about it: that I'm probably just deeply tired and my mind and body are taking some deep rest. For the first few years, I'd feel like I was going right to sleep sitting up. I was exhausted and my body and mind needed to take the rest they required, and this was a way to get it. I was so thirsty for quiet and rest! Rather than it interfering with my sleep, by keeping it to 20 minutes in the early morning and 20 minutes in the afternoon, I found meditation to be a saviour – it wasn't taking away my sleep-appetite: instead it was helping me to replenish my energy throughout the day, feel more clear-headed in my thinking, less stressed, and more relaxed come sleep time. I also found practising meditation made me less reactive to ambient noise:

I learned to relax and let the sounds wash over me, so it became easier to tune out noises or noisy thoughts and drop off to sleep more easily. I found that I could stay asleep more easily, because small noises in the night no longer disturbed me in the times when I'd be closer to the surface of waking up.

Gently guiding the wandering mind back to a chosen focus is one of the main keys to the meditation process. Meditation seems to train the brain to have thoughts and not allow them to cause distress, but to come back to centre and enter a relaxed state. This can prove very helpful when the mind experiences a stream of thoughts at sleep time.

How to meditate

1 Using a word, mantra, or your breath, focus your attention on it in a relaxed way, without gripping on to it; just bring it into your mind.

2 When other thoughts intrude (and they will), let them do this without resisting them, but also, once you realise your mind has wandered, just bring your attention back to the focus you chose, remembering that you can laugh at yourself if you get frustrated and start judging or criticising yourself for having a thought.

Here are two classic ways of approaching meditation: through focusing on your breath or focusing on a repeated syllable.

SIMPLE BREATH MEDITATION TECHNIQUE: INTERNAL AWARENESS

One approach is to become mindful of your breath without controlling or manipulating it. Unlike the breathing practices in Step 2, you are just watching what your breath is doing naturally. This 'mindfulness of breathing' is used in Buddhist meditation as

Group practice

When you practise meditation, of course you can do it alone. However, you can gain a lot from being with an experienced meditation teacher or meditating in a group; attunement occurs. It is very rare in our society that we encounter people with a calm, relaxed nervous system, who have trained their bodies and minds to enter a peaceful state in general, and to go into deep relaxation at will. If your meditation teacher is practising regularly, they will have a sense about them that is different to other people when they enter a room, and even at their most agitated they will have the ability to regulate their nervous system and to come back to balance easily. Meditating in a group, when many people enter a relaxed state all together, can be incredibly powerful: you are surrounded by others who are relaxed, breathing slowly, and there is often a palpable sense of steadiness in the room. While at first, for me, I always felt like the fidgety one, I did slowly learn to settle, entraining with the group over time.

While this can be explained in spiritual terms, I also like to think of it in terms of our modern understanding of *mirror neurons*, which enable us to pick up on the states of others through neurophysiological means. Think of the way a child senses the calm or distress of its caregivers – we develop in ways that relate to the physical and mental states of those around us because they give us powerful cues that we might need for survival.

Just as a highly stressed person's state ripples off of them and affects others in the room even without that person saying a word, a calm, relaxed and spacious person can have a strong influence on you. A person who embodies this very strongly, and a room full of people in this state, are very powerful stabilising forces as you learn to sit and turn your attention inward.

well as Western-based mindfulness programmes. You will feel different sensations caused by the movements of your breath in your body. The technique is a small variation on the two basic steps in 'How to Meditate' on page 139.

◆ Sit quietly and comfortably, unmoving but not forcing yourself to sit so still that you feel tense.
◆ Bring your attention to the sensation of your breath as it enters your nose, particularly inside the nostrils, where there is a bit of moisture in the mucus membrane.
◆ Begin by noticing the temperature, texture and quality of the air moving in and out of your nose.
◆ Stay with this awareness and when your mind goes elsewhere, gently bring it back to the inside of the nose.
◆ Observe your breath without altering your inhalation or exhalation, noticing the 'arising and passing' of the breath as well the thoughts moving through.
◆ Stay here for between 10 and 20 minutes and do this as a regular practice.

This is particularly useful if you have a tendency towards overwhelming thoughts when you're trying to get to sleep – slowing down your mind, creating a more spacious awareness. It has the ability to begin calming your nervous system effectively and quickly, shifting from beta to alpha brainwaves.

MANTRA MEDITATION TECHNIQUE

Using a mantra for meditation is a widespread and long-established practice in the West. In meditation, mantra doesn't mean 'life philosophy' or 'affirmation'. It is a simple syllable or phrase that you repeat inwardly, over and over in your mind, without grasping on to it, forcing your mind to repeat it or shouting it into your brain.

The word mantra has two syllables – 'man' comes from *manas*,

App, video or teacher?

Many traditional meditation lineages involve a teacher giving a practice or mantra to the student. I do recommend that if at all possible you get yourself a real, live meditation teacher or go to a class with a seasoned meditator leading it. While phone apps or online tutorials or recordings can be helpful for reminding you to meditate, serve as a timer and offer you encouraging words or music, there is no substitute for a living, heart-beating, breathing presence in the room with you.

meaning 'mind', and 'tra' from *traverse*, meaning 'to move across'. You can think of a mantra as a vehicle that holds or carries your mind, and you hold it lightly, directing your mind back to it when thoughts, sensations and emotions come up.

I was given one that I have used for years; it's not used for anything other than meditation, and it's not an English word, so my mind has no other associations with it than 'it's time to meditate'. Much like Pavlov's dogs, who learned that a certain bell tone was associated with being fed, and would salivate upon hearing the bell, when I think my mantra, my mind gets ready for meditation.

As I mentioned before, the embodied state of the teacher in the room is one reason to learn from a trained meditation teacher; another is that s/he can give you a mantra based on your mind and its needs, rather than a one size fits all. Clearly, sounds have different qualities, and repeating one sound will have a different effect on you than repeating another. There is even a belief that different constitutional types need different mantras for their balancing effects. Having some informed guidance can be helpful.

The Transcendental Meditation/Vedic Meditation method has a strong evidence base, pointing out its effectiveness for reducing stress and overcoming sleep problems. After many years of doing my yoga and breathing practices before bed, which helped me to get to sleep and stay asleep, when I was ready to learn properly to meditate and practised it regularly, the quality of my sleep improved dramatically.

The practice usually involves receiving a mantra from the teacher, and once initiated into its use, you use this same mantra to meditate for 20 minutes twice a day. This seems like a lot at first, but when you think about how long you might take flicking through social media or checking emails, or compared with tossing and turning for hours in bed, it's not that much. I found that it really just required me to set aside the time, and to plan it in.

Learning and practising yoga postures and breathing exercises for a while made it easier for me to sit and meditate than if I'd tried it cold: I needed to learn to sit and settle. I'd always been a fidgety person! I do know other people who can stumble right into a meditation practice and do it immediately but find the body stretches or breathing practices harder. Either way is fine.

The key is regularity, and to make it a priority. Traditionally, the first practice is done in the morning before the day's activity kicks in, and the second in the afternoon, before the evening meal. The commitment and focus that meditation brings helps to regulate sleep by having profound effects at two essential times of the day: when you first wake up, and in the mid-afternoon slump.

As you meditate during these key times, you may notice that you have different flavours of meditation. For example, you may have a very active meditation with a ton of thoughts: you can regard this as a clearing or 'purification' within your meditation, allowing thoughts to arise, be digested and cleared out. Or, you may have a sense that you are actually falling asleep in your meditation, in which case your body and mind are getting some deep, replenishing rest. Neither is wrong, and both can be very helpful for you: we need both when seeking to repair our sleep. You can trust that the thing your body and mind need most is what you will get!

HOW TO DO MANTRA MEDITATION

- Sit comfortably for a moment.
- Begin with the intention to think a simple syllable (the mantra). If you want one that is simple to remember, use: HREEM. It will generally hold no associations in your mind, which is exactly the point of this mantra.
- Bring the mantra into the mind; when the mind wanders, bring the mantra back in.
- Do this without setting a timer. If you are curious about how much time has passed, look at your watch or clock.
- After 20 minutes have passed, take a two- to three-minute 'buffer' without the mantra, in order to return to regular waking consciousness.

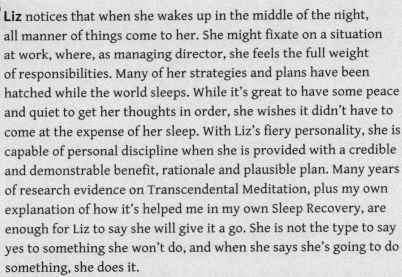

CASE STUDY

Liz notices that when she wakes up in the middle of the night, all manner of things come to her. She might fixate on a situation at work, where, as managing director, she feels the full weight of responsibilities. Many of her strategies and plans have been hatched while the world sleeps. While it's great to have some peace and quiet to get her thoughts in order, she wishes it didn't have to come at the expense of her sleep. With Liz's fiery personality, she is capable of personal discipline when she is provided with a credible and demonstrable benefit, rationale and plausible plan. Many years of research evidence on Transcendental Meditation, plus my own explanation of how it's helped me in my own Sleep Recovery, are enough for Liz to say she will give it a go. She is not the type to say yes to something she won't do, and when she says she's going to do something, she does it.

We look together at her daily schedule, and identify two periods in which she can do a 20-minute meditation. The first is on her morning train commute. Even if she drives into work, she can park her car at the park near her office, and in good weather meditate on a bench. On gloomy or rainy days, she finds a quiet parking spot, gets

Research has shown meditation to have these effects: feeling calmer throughout the day, reduced cortisol (the 'stress hormone'), normalised blood pressure, decreased risk of heart attack and stroke, lessening of anxiety and depression, and improvement in brain function and memory. All of these contribute towards better-quality sleep and decrease insomnia because they de-stress your body and retrain your brain to let go and get some sleep, making you feel generally more sane and sorted.

out of the driver's seat and sits on the passenger side, locks the doors, rolls up the windows, and closes her eyes there. After work, she has made a plan with her husband and children that she will say hello, go directly up to her room for 20 minutes, meditate and then come back down to greet the family and begin the evening.

During this time, she 'burns through' thoughts and the events of the day, usually in the first 10–15 minutes of the meditation. Over time, she's noticed that she seems to settle for at least a few minutes into a state of rest and calm, and often has a creative thought or memory bubble to the surface.

Liz finds that these buffers at the start and end of her working day leave her refreshed, focused and more present – first for meeting the challenges of a demanding job, and then allowing the working day to be dissolved so that it doesn't bleed into family time, and she's more present for her family. She's noticed that, at bedtime, she's less likely to encounter the parade of thoughts , wakes less in the night for problem solving, and usually now wakes in the middle of the night only when she has had a glass of wine with dinner.

STEP 4

Restore a sense of calm

WHEN LIFE FEELS HARMONIOUS and truly resolved, we often have an easier time sleeping. I know that when I feel conflicted, unsure, resentful, fearful, angry, sad or any other negative emotion, I can lose sleep more easily. Of course, when I feel joyful or elated, and excited by life, I can also stay up late, but it's for good reasons, so I don't tend to mind so much! Rather than focusing on the amount of sleep I get, I've learned to focus on the quality of sleep and, more importantly, my physical and mental state during the day – and I encourage you to do this as well. This step will help you to manage upset, both in the moment and in the longer term, so that you can not only get some better rest, but feel more resolved.

While yoga, breathing, meditation and the other tools in this programme do help us to find peace and calm, sometimes life circumstances stir us up. This step in your Sleep Recovery involves soothing yourself and letting go as well as learning to work through difficult emotions.

Part 1 is a lot like soothing a baby who's overwhelmed: sometimes we need to settle down, let strong feelings dissipate and calm ourselves. In doing this, we *change* our internal experience, shifting away from the anger, sadness or other difficult emotions. This is a good set of skills to have, as it helps restore peace in the moment – either before sleep, during a mid-night wake-up or throughout the day. This step also enables you to develop another important skill: that of working-through. If we don't *experience* difficult emotions and move *through* them, we can stay gripped by them.

Part 2 looks at insomnia that arises from life events that are not merely emotional, but are truly terrifying, overwhelming or life-threatening. When we have experiences that send us into shock, the after-effects may range from a state of high-level panic to a low-grade but chronic hyper-alertness that lasts for a very long time. Sometimes the shock effects go away on their own, but they may need to be released through some specifically focused therapeutic work. Many people who come for Sleep Recovery are not aware of the extent to which they are suffering from a post-traumatic reaction, and what to do about it. This section will enable you to determine whether this may be part of your problem and offers some tools and ideas about where to find help if you need it.

PART 1:
EMOTIONAL SORTING-OUT

My students and clients are always quick to volunteer information about their coffee intake, their bedtimes and wake times and many details of their daily habits. But scratch beneath the surface a bit, and often something else emerges: they're going through a divorce, have lost a loved one recently, are having arguments with someone important to them, their company's being restructured and work feels like a minefield, or deadlines and productivity pressures are mounting. If we look at it on paper, it seems clear that an emotionally volatile or difficult situation can affect our sleep, but in the midst of the maelstrom it's hard to recognise what's happening. Unresolved situations – sometimes current and sometimes long past – arouse powerful feelings that come to call in the quiet hours.

One of the most common causes of insomnia is a life event that interrupts your sleep for some reason. While some of these are purely logistical in that they ask us to keep a different schedule, some events can create a high level of stress or involve an emotional 'trigger'. Changing jobs, a relationship breakdown/breakup, moving to a new place or a change in living situation, the birth of a child or a change to the family composition, loss of income or savings, the death of a loved one: family, friend, colleague or pet. One woman in her 30s, the mother of a small child, had slept really well both before and after the birth of her daughter, but three sessions into our work, she revealed that her sleep problems had begun after she found out that her husband was having an affair. Without recognising the emotionally charged situation for what it was, and dealing with it internally and in her relationship, the breathing, yoga practices and meditation didn't stand much of a chance on their own in getting her back into balance.

Some events may not seem as personally catastrophic as the ones above, but even events that aren't happening to you directly, or that seem minor at the time, can remind you of other painful experiences, directly or indirectly. I have said to myself about certain things, 'I don't know why this bothers me so much!' While it may seem strange, we can be affected at a deep level by things that seem inconsequential at first. Sometimes we're wrung out or tense, but don't know why. It's as if what we don't want to or can't feel during the day are the monsters under the bed that come creeping out when we shut the lights off. Tension or physical pain, or repetitive thoughts, can all signal the same thing: I'm upset. I recall going to a meal with friends and finding myself tense and anxious, and it wasn't until I used the emotional release technique I'll tell you about in this step (see page 154) that I could pinpoint how I felt and what was bothering me. Without that practice, I'd probably have stayed tense all day and gone to bed subtly upset without understanding why – and without letting it go.

Something powerful happens if we can stay with what's bothering us and tolerate strong feelings: they tend to subside and we can better work out what's driving those feelings. Often, difficult or painful emotions tell us that some situation needs resolution; it's said that true wisdom is in knowing the difference between the situations that can be changed, and the ones that can't. Sometimes working through means having a difficult conversation and speaking up about something that's not right, making an apology, or reframing a past situation that can only be changed by recognising how we allow it to affect us today.

Living with unhealed emotional trauma is a bit like walking around on a fractured bone: although you can't see the wound, you

Beneath the surface

Most people feel they should be 'over' difficult life events or transitions in a phenomenally short space of time. I am always sad to see people put so much pressure on themselves to move on from pain or change. I remember that at the height of my own insomnia I was working at a very stressful job – in a part of the Manhattan crime prosecutor's office that dealt with some pretty horrible stuff. As I look back on that time, it makes perfect sense that my sleep was disturbed: every day I saw things that most people only ever see in fictional form on television cop shows, and Monday through Friday were filled with atrocities that made me feel incredibly unsafe walking around New York. Of course, consciously I thought I was tough and could handle it, but my fears came out in my (lack of) sleep and frightened dreams. It was only years later that I put two and two together: unconscious fear was zapping my sleep. I've since learned that a lot of police officers, firefighters and others exposed to danger and violence have trouble sleeping – and it makes perfect sense to me now.

can definitely feel the pain and you'll need professional help to heal it. Since trauma responses can cause some of our longest-term sleeplessness, it's vital to get the help you need to start feeling safer at a deep, creaturely level. I'll give you some examples and suggestions for trauma-related insomnia and healing the longer-term emotional causes of your sleepless nights.

Instead of only dealing with the symptoms, we'll try to get to the cause of emotional sleeplessness. If there are emotional roots to your sleep problems, using the DIY tools here will help you on the road to better rest now, and you can flag up some areas where you may want to work with a qualified counsellor or psychotherapist to do some emotional housekeeping.

What am I feeling?

Clearly, some emotions feel good while others feel awful; some stir us up and others settle us down. It's completely natural to feel all of the basic human emotions, even the ones we don't like: fear, anger, sadness, grief, anxiety, shame, resentment or loneliness.

Activation

tense   alert

nervous   excited

stressed   elated

upset   happy

Unpleasant   **Pleasant**

sad   contented

depressed   serene

bored   relaxed

fatigued   calm

Deactivation

We may have different ways of knowing how we feel. I have one client who regularly feels a choking sensation in his throat when he is angry, one who feels a stabbing pain in her stomach when she is anxious, and one who starts to collapse and feel exhausted when she feels ashamed. If you can recognise your own emotional signals, you can move the sensation of tension or collapse through your body. This helps you to discern more clearly when a life situation is affecting you so that you can clear it up and move on, and in the process restore your ability to rest at ease.

Shifting states

If I'm getting tense during the day, I'll often get up and stretch out my shoulders, or do a forward bend, take a walk or practise some deep breaths because I want to shift my state from one that feels bad to one that feels good. Yoga and mindful practices do this in a healthy way, while other ways of shifting our state can sabotage our sleep by creating more drama in our lives or by altering our brain chemistry and physical state in unhelpful ways. Plus, not dealing with what's really bothering us runs the risk that we add to a seeping swamp of backlogged and unresolved resentments, pent-up anger, unprocessed grief or stultifying shame. So, while we may need things to change the way we feel in the moment, we also tend to rest more easily when we clear out the backlog.

Doing the practices in Step 1 help you to shift your energy, mind and your emotions through moving your body. You can also take a moment to change your thinking to shift your emotions: calling to mind positive experiences can be very constructive in the short term. If you can do this, it can have an immediate and powerful effect on how you feel in the moment. One practice that has become popular in positive psychology is writing a gratitude list.

I've done this frequently: first, I move my body to release tension, then I sit to write a list of 10 things I'm grateful for. I call to mind people, places and experiences that I appreciate, and that make me feel good. They can be really simple or very profound, from a gorgeous morning coffee with a sea view, to the feel of mud under my boots during a walk in my favourite local park, to the appreciation I have for a close friendship with my mother. With each thing I'm grateful for, I try to feel it physically, recalling the sensory experience: the scene, the place where I feel it in my body, and even a scent or taste.

I start by writing down something I'm grateful for or really appreciate and in as much detail as possible: I really appreciate the feeling of walking through Hampstead Heath on a grey morning when the air is crisp, it's uncrowded and silent. Then I notice what I can see, feel in my body, smell, taste and touch. I love how the cold air chills my nose, and the damp misty rain makes my cheeks flush pink and warm. I love the scent of the leaves and the boggy smell of the mud. I love the way my feet stay dry in my woolly socks tucked into waterproof Wellington boots, so that I can hear the slurping sound of the mud as I trundle up little hills. I notice the snap of twigs under my feet, and the million shades of green in the thick wooded maze-like parts of the park that make me feel wealthy on a soul level. When I think of this, and focus on these sensations, I feel my shoulders soften, my heart rate slows down, and I breathe more easily, just from shifting my attention, or experiencing a different feeling in the moment.

Sometimes I even call to mind situations that were initially difficult, from which I had to learn something new. I felt so good when the difficult part was over! This includes feeling grateful for my years of sleepless nights – because these gave me the kick that I needed to start talking about what was bothering me, and learn all the techniques I've amassed for this book.

Gratitude and appreciation

Write out what you're grateful for, immersing yourself in the sensory experiences of each. Be as specific as you can, using your imagination to mine the richness of the full experience.

1 Use this prompt:

I'm grateful for

or

I really appreciate

2 Then fill in the sensory experience:

When I think of this, I can recall this scene:

The feeling in my body is:

The tastes and smells are:

The sounds I can hear are:

Do this as fully as you can for between five and ten things.

Emotional body cleansing

While it's great to change our attention so that we feel better in the moment, it's also important to be able to sit with difficult emotions so that we can gain insight into what's really bothering us. I once heard, and believe, this saying: What you resist will persist. We can only temporarily shunt difficult emotions to the side; eventually we need to deal with the real feelings and seek resolution, or the emotional gremlins will tend to keep popping up from under the bed and grabbing us!

Getting to the emotional root of tension in the body, and breathing through it, letting it 'arise and pass', can help us to gain insight and to ease into sleep more deeply. This next practice helps focus on the areas of the body where you hold tension, and acknowledge and release any associated emotions.

EMOTIONAL RELEASE MEDITATION: STEP BY STEP

* Sit upright, comfortably, with your eyes closed, and breathe gently for 30 seconds or so. Become aware of your body, noticing the chair or floor, feeling your feet, your legs, hips, back and arms.
* Feel the place in your body where you're holding the most tension. There may be more than one place. Pick the one that is the most tense, or the most attention-grabbing. Don't worry about getting it wrong. You can choose one area, and go back for another area later. For example: I notice a heat and tightness in my throat.
* Ask yourself what feeling or *tone* is associated with that tightness. You may be able to sense that it feels like impatience, anxiety, fear, anger or sadness. For example: The sensation of tightness in my throat feels *angry*.
* Breathe with awareness in the area, noticing the sensation there.

* Say to yourself (in your head), as you inhale, 'I feel x', and then insert for x whatever the feeling is. For example: 'I feel angry' or 'I feel the anger'.

* On your exhale (and this is the revolutionary part), you say to yourself, again in your head, 'I welcome x' or 'I accept x' or 'I allow x', and put in that same emotion. For example: 'I welcome the anger' or 'I allow the anger to be there'.

* As you do this, keep breathing, keep noticing the feeling in the area, and notice if the sensation changes, and what the feeling is along with the new sensation. Notice any changes in the sensation and in the emotion you associate with it. Most often, you will notice that the sensation and emotion will increase, then change, and eventually decrease if you stay with it. For example: The anger has changed, it now feels like heaviness or sadness in my throat.

* When the emotion shifts, the sensation may diminish or change location. For example: The tightness and the heaviness in my throat have softened, and now I feel a heaviness in my heart.

* If the sensation changes location, stay with that area until you have felt into and allowed the shift to occur there. For example: I feel the heaviness in my heart and tears start to form in my eyes. I recall a memory of a person I love who has died, and as I have some tears, I feel a sense of release. The tightness has gone, and I realise I miss my friend.

Many people tell me this helps them build insight into the link between their body sensation and emotional state, and that this practice leaves them feeling freer and clearer. You may start out agitated and angry and then release into a softer emotion. At other times, you may feel collapsed and drained, only to release the emotion and feel energy return to your body. Try it a few times in different situations. I find that the release of pent-up or unconscious emotion often allows sleep to arrive more readily, and enables me to sleep more deeply.

See drama: keep driving

I take a group of students on a retreat in Greece each summer. Every time I take the two-hour drive from the city of Thessaloniki down to a little port town, I pass a highway sign listing the towns off of the exit. It says: Drama 5km. I laugh to myself and make the same joke: see Drama in the distance, and keep driving! The concept of the 'drama triangle' from a branch of psychology called Transactional Analysis can be incredibly helpful here in sorting out conflicts you keep turning over in your mind before bed. When you're thinking some disturbing or repetitive thought, it can be useful to ask: Which one of these roles am I taking on – the victim, the rescuer, or the persecutor?

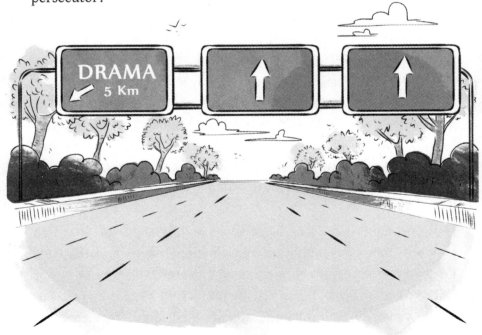

The victim or the wronged might say:	The persecutor or the justice-seeker might say:	The rescuer or the saviour might say:
They did something bad to me!	'How dare they!'	I can fix it.
It's my fault.	They should be punished.	I should have done more.
How could they do this to me?	They were wrong.	How can I make it better?
Why does this always happen to me?	I can't believe they did this.	How can I help?
That should never have happened.	I am right.	Oh, poor you!
It's just not fair.	I'll show them.	
Poor me...	I need to get revenge.	

Each of these positions is trying to make sense of a situation or take control of it in a way that assumes too much or not enough responsibility. If you tend to get stuck in any of these ways of thinking, you may be trying to do things for other people or to pass responsibility on to others in a way that will ultimately sabotage your health and well-being. It's easy to get caught in any one of these positions when we are upset about something and, like a dog worrying a bone, it's hard for us to let go of being 'right' in whatever way we have thought about a situation.

However, it's only when we look at things from a range of perspectives, and step OUT of the triangle of feeling like we've been wronged, that we have to avenge, or that we have to 'fix it' that we can get some perspective. Our thoughts usually follow our emotions – none of which are wrong – but finding a way through a situation that doesn't create more drama requires that we step out of the position we're in.

Work it out: communication for clarity

I used to think I was the only one whose head was filled with unresolved conflicts turning over and over in my mind, getting in the way of my sleep or waking me in the middle of the night. Since working with many others on their sleep, I've found that this is a very common problem, and that in order to minimise emotionally driven insomnia, we need tools to meet our emotional needs and resolve the situations that plague us. We can think of this as a kind of emotional housekeeping, and it can really help to clear up long-term sleeplessness.

Emotional insomnia doesn't have to be prompted by extreme situations, but can be the result of backlogged unexpressed sentiments or resentments. Being upset with someone or with a situation can mean it turns over and over in your head like a stone in a rock-tumbler; it can be like a heavy weight on your chest, or set an angry fire in your belly.

The advice given to my grandmother's generation was 'never go to bed mad': in other words, try to resolve your conflicts before going to sleep. Throughout their marriage of more than 60 years, my grandparents believed in communicating and resolving conflicts or upsets before bedtime.

Over time, resentments and conflicts can lead to emotional distress, physical tension, mental turmoil and sleeplessness. Doing your emotional housekeeping – pursuing harmony in the emotional realm, learning ways to resolve emotional friction – helps us to rest free of tension and with a clear conscience. In fact, an essential part of many addiction recovery programmes, where people are seeking to put down drugs, alcohol, gambling or other self-sabotaging behaviour, is to take stock of long-held and daily resentments, take responsibility for their own feelings and recognise the damaging behaviours that are ways of acting out to get away from fear, guilt, shame and other reactions.

There are countless techniques you can use to help you identify and deal with emotions and conflicts, and trained counsellors or therapists will have a range of skills and tools to share with you. I recommend a method to my clients, and where I've been able to practise it in my own life, I've found it immensely useful: it's called non-violent communication.

It starts with getting clear on our own emotions, then looking at the situation that has sparked the feelings, and finally getting clear about what we would like to feel instead and how to get there. This enables us to take steps to meet our own needs: negotiate with others to help us or recognise that a situation will not be resolved in a way that meets our needs, so we can step away or make change. It's particularly useful to do after the previous exercises, so that you know what's going in inside yourself before taking action with other people.

Even when we can't change the external situation, it can be useful to realise that we do have the power to change our way of dealing with it. There's a popular saying that I like, in which we ask to be given the serenity to accept what we can't change, the courage to

What is non-violent communication?

A technique for conflict resolution called 'non-violent communication' (NVC) sees conflicts between people as arising because we fail to communicate about, and meet, our human needs in ways that work, and we misunderstand or disregard others' needs. When we feel pain or discomfort, especially in relation to other people's actions, too often we use coercive or manipulative language that makes other people feel what *we* don't want to feel: blamed, afraid, guilty or ashamed, to name just a few. Learning to communicate in ways that respect all involved in a situation can be a key to feeling clearer and resting easier. There are great online tutorials and readily available books by Marshall Rosenberg, the pioneer of NVC, and others.

change what we can, and the wisdom to know the difference. You can think of it as an appeal to your own deepest wisdom, a prayer, or a way of connecting to a perspective far broader than the part of you that's become locked in a difficult or emotive situation.

Doing our emotional housekeeping means we clarify our needs, our feelings, our perceptions and our requests, and although we can't avoid conflict, we can minimise it and deal with it more effectively when it comes up. If you maintain a regular practice of emotional housekeeping, you know that there will be a way out of difficult situations, and it's easier to put whatever is bothering you down before you put your head on the pillow at night.

PART 2:
DE-TRAUMATISE YOUR SLEEP

Even if at one point you enjoyed healthy, satisfying sleep, a traumatic event can destabilise this. To recover your sleep, you'll need to relearn how to find the relaxed state you once knew. If, on the other hand, you can't remember a time when you had pleasant, restful sleep, and it's never been a refuge but a burden, this may be down to feeling unsafe in an earlier stage of life: if you were exposed to danger, risk or abuse, you might – consciously or unconsciously – be afraid of going sleep. If this has been your experience, your Sleep Recovery may involve setting up an entirely new set of experiences – creating new mental and physical resources.

When I initially started my yoga practice years ago, some activities that were supposed to be relaxing – meditation or mindfulness, relaxation techniques and some yoga moves – instead of chilling me out had the opposite effect. For me, meditation was the hardest, not just because I couldn't concentrate, but because I closed my eyes and not only did the ticking clock across the room feel like it was right beside my ear, but I felt a deep fear and panic that I couldn't explain. I kept with it, received a lot of encouragement and instruction, sat with teachers in classes, and built a sense of safety. If you find yourself drifting off and checking out, if you have illogical resistance to certain movements or find it difficult to close your eyes and relax, you're not alone: in any yoga class of more than 10 people, I find that at least one student may be unable to do the part where you lie down on your back in stillness at the end. Some people may be deeply uncomfortable with breath practices, or may find it disconcerting to shut their eyes to try meditation in a roomful of people. In bigger groups, I can see a handful of people who have reactions like fidgeting or spacing-out, or being 'unable to relax'.

Several years ago, a woman in her late 20s came to my weekly yoga class; she loved yoga and was very attentive and engaged. After a few weeks, I noticed that every so often she'd be a few moves behind the rest of the class, a bit spaced-out, with her eyes floating up to the ceiling. After class one day, I checked in with her to say I'd noticed she seemed to go somewhere at different points during the class and wondered if she was okay. Over time, we realised that poses involving lying on her back with her legs open would set off the reaction: when a past trauma was *triggered* she would dissociate, or disconnect her mind from her body. This is something I have since learned is not uncommon with people who have suffered abuse in early life (and so the approach to practices needs to be tailored appropriately).

Some signs of post-traumatic stress can show up in your sleep: a sudden startle or surge of fear just as you are about to 'let go' and fall asleep, nightmares or night terrors, or waking with a racing heart in a panic state. If, along with your sleep problems, you're also experiencing anxiety, phobias or unexplained fears, severe mood swings, hyper-vigilance, obsessions/compulsions, physical symptoms that seem to have no medical diagnosis – for example, a chronic pain – or difficulty with learning and concentration, you may be experiencing post-traumatic insomnia.

While some people stay up late and avoid sleep because they are overworking or feel anxious about sleep, there is also a possibility that we can stay up too late and stay away from sleep because it feels unsafe or makes us too vulnerable. When you sabotage your sleep in this way, it can be a sign that you are consciously or unconsciously *afraid* to go to sleep. I experienced this for a time, and some of my clients identify with it as well. You may *know* what you 'should' do, but your sleep habits are consistently sabotaged, sometimes by addictive or compulsive actions. Tina, a woman in her late 40s whose story appears at the end of this step, was so afraid of her lifelong nightmares, and so afraid to go to sleep, that she would drink alcohol or take sedatives to get to sleep, or stay awake long into the night watching movies or TV. Even though these habits sabotaged her sleep, they would temporarily numb her out, so that she wouldn't feel anxious about going to bed. Coping mechanisms like these don't repair the underlying *cause* of the insomnia; they stop working quickly, and often have detrimental effects on your physical and mental state the next day.

WHAT CAN CAUSE TRAUMATIC SHOCK AND POST-TRAUMATIC INSOMNIA?

An attack, physical injury or accident, war, natural disaster, birth trauma, severe abandonment, torture or abuse can cause strong reactions. We'll look at three forms of post-trauma reaction – PTSD, developmental trauma and 'complex' PTSD – and offer you some suggestions for an approach to post-traumatic Sleep Recovery.

Shocking or overwhelming events have an impact on us as we mature through the stages of development – from infancy, childhood and adolescence into adulthood. Neglect and abandonment can cause disruptions in a child's development, and abuse within the family at an early age can get in the way of forming a secure attachment to others. A child hospitalised at an early age for prolonged periods may lose some of her sense of earlier successful attachment. A child who's been in danger during times of rest or sleep may never have learned to rest comfortably and to relax enough to sleep well. These all affect the basic sense of security and safety, which affects our nervous system and can cause a post-traumatic stress response.

We now understand how humans' and wild animals' biological response systems are activated in response to perceived life-threatening situations. When we're overwhelmed by a threat where fight or flight isn't possible, we get into a freeze response. Whereas animals will shake or run away, which helps to dissipate the stress hormones and tension in their bodies so they can re-establish a balance, we often tamp down our instinctive body responses, which effectively traps the stress in our bodies, and so we can stay in a highly charged yet frozen state, much like a car with both the brakes and the accelerator floored simultaneously.

We get stopped by overwhelming situations. When our nervous system hasn't been able to complete the process of orienting us to our surroundings by fighting or running away – in other words, if it gets blocked from doing what it needs to do – we can get stuck in one of two emotional states: rage, which is the urge to fight that's been frustrated, or a very physical sense of terror panic, which happens if we are blocked from running away. We can hold in our bodies and our emotions a sense of traumatic anxiety when we have had to bottle up or restrain.

Basically, if you've been broadsided by a shock, your body–mind system can stay on high alert to protect you from harm. This makes sense when there is danger present, but post-trauma disorders mean that the alarm bells are always switched on, or that they switch on in response to cues that spark a memory or sensory cue: a specific sight, sound or smell can spark a flashback or provoke a bodily response. What may seem like 'nothing' to one person may be of great importance to a person with a trauma response. It gets tricky because sometimes, long after the fact, we don't recognise that the physical sensation is there when we have an emotional response.

If you've been through a traumatic event, your body's response to it can actually recondition your nervous system, so when you do get to sleep it can be far less restful than it should be: increased arousal in your nervous system will continue *during* sleep as well as when you're awake, so it may take you longer to fall asleep, you may be highly sensitive to noise, or you might awaken more frequently during the night than you did before. Of course, this means that sleep isn't really enjoyable, so if this is the case you may be self-restricting your sleep, meaning you'll want to do everything else but sleep and stay up long into the night with distractions, because going to bed can simply feel too frustrating.

HOW TO REPAIR POST-TRAUMATIC INSOMNIA

If you've experienced a trauma, Somatic Experiencing (a method for completing the fight/flight response 'frozen' in the body) and other types of work with a qualified therapist can guide you gently into the realm of body sensation and help you to regulate your own nervous system by tracking the subtle body experience and sensation, *gently and bit by bit,* letting the involuntary releases of tension – and often the emotions – happen. Recovery from trauma-based insomnia relies on you either relearning or re-patterning your response to sleep and relaxation, or learning for the first time (as in the case of very early trauma) the capacity to self-soothe. In addition to discharging the hyper-alert, heightened state, it's also important to *repair* the sense of safety or establish it for the first time. When we learn to create feelings of safety and comfort, this decreases the urge to escape, numb or self-medicate that spurs sleep-sabotaging habits such as alcohol and drug abuse, and other addictive behaviours that can cause insomnia or make it worse.

Working together with a therapist can help you re-establish or develop a core within yourself in which you feel secure, creating a 'resource' for safety, rather than attaching to things, people or substances outside of yourself to create that sense of safety. This sense of security then extends into your sleep patterns, making it easier to release into sleep and helping you to feel, at a very deep level, *secure* enough to stay asleep.

Since shock trauma causes a physiological, biologically natural response, its effect is not under mental, logical-rational control, so talk-based counselling or psychotherapy may not totally resolve the symptoms. If you can find a qualified therapist who is trained and established in a method like Somatic Experiencing, you might find this helps you to recover from the psychological and physiological effects of trauma more effectively, as body, mind and emotions are all addressed together. Exploring trauma-sensitive yoga – a way of adapting yoga principles for healing specific PTSD symptoms – can also be helpful, as it's more specifically geared towards developing the internal capacity to feel your responses to movement and create a sense of personal safety and ability to act on your own behalf. If you're interested in more information, take a look at the resources at the end of this book. One of the reasons this Sleep Recovery programme works well for people with trauma symptoms is that it teaches you to calm your nervous system and gives you a sense of agency over your own body: an ability to manage your tension and relaxation yourself.

Post-traumatic insomnnia: what to look for

Things you might experience after a trauma	How yoga helps with healing
HYPER-AROUSAL: When we're alarmed and startled, our heart rate and breath rate increase, and we start to sweat.	Bringing gentle attention to, and eventually slowing down, the rate of your breathing can increase your sense of safety. Slowly increase the length of your exhale: the ability to do this grows over time, and becomes a vital resource to soothe and calm you if you feel activated or triggered. Loosening up your muscles with yoga stretches will help you to feel more mentally calm and balanced.
CONSTRICTION OR TIGHTENING-UP: This happens when our perception narrows. Our internal organs constrict and our digestive system is inhibited.	To counter narrowing and tightening, which our bodies do as a way to protect us from danger, we can start to breathe more deeply, and to move slowly with a sense of internal rhythm that feels easy and expansive. Pressing outwards with your arms and legs to lengthen your muscles can help you feel a sense of space and release. Gentle torso- and spine-twisting postures can also bring greater movement around your abdomen and help you to release the muscles used for breathing and around your ribcage, shoulders and neck.

Things you might experience after a trauma	How yoga helps with healing
CHECKING-OUT OR GOING NUMB, ALSO CALLED DISSOCIATION: A way that human beings can release endorphins ('nature's internal opium') that numb the pain associated with attack. Endorphins can help us to endure experiences we may not otherwise be able to bear. This can lead to a feeling of 'fragmentation', in which part of the body becomes disconnected from awareness or goes numb. You may have had an experience of feeling separate from, or outside of, yourself.	Connecting what you see, what you feel physically, and movement can help you to reconnect with your body – to find the parts that have got a bit lost. Yoga stretches that couple movement with breath awareness help you to focus on body sensation as you move. For example, watching your foot stepping back or touching the active body area in a yoga pose with your hand can help your brain to reconnect to the physical sensation, e.g. pressing your hand on to the back of your thigh as you stretch there.
DENIAL OR SHOCK: Not knowing how you're feeling or if something's wrong. Being 'in denial' is not something we do intentionally. Shock is a state of overwhelm in which we're not able to take in something frightening or life-threatening that has occurred.	Conscious movement and breath can take you back to the present moment – when you're 'here', you can better acknowledge what you feel. When you are able to soothe yourself instead of checking out, you can better explore the past events to heal them.
FEELINGS OF HELPLESSNESS: Being unable to move or freezing up.	Moving your body at your own will, making different shapes and gaining strength can help you to feel more in your body and enable you to act on your own behalf. Some self-directed movement can help you to tolerate stronger experiences before tuning out, so you become more conscious, process emotions and release them.

Tina wished she could just 'find the right button to press' to make the nightmares stop. She drank at least one bottle of red wine every night, which sometimes kept her from dreaming – meaning she could avoid the terrifying nightmares that made her dread sleep. She had a hangover most mornings, and she had trouble remembering things.

Tina had tried many solutions for her sleep, which cost her a small fortune, and still she suffered. She liked the idea of yoga, but wouldn't attend a group class because even *thinking* about lying down on a yoga mat in a room full of strangers made her nervous: if her body relaxed even a little bit, she would convulse and tighten up in a spasm, which embarrassed her. I've learned that if people have the type of symptoms Tina has, there can be some kind of abuse or other trust-based trauma in their history. She was already in therapy, and came to me for *yoga therapy* focusing on sleep, so my remit was clear: there were things I didn't ask, and we kept to the yoga on its own. Rather than committing to a whole pack of classes, she worked with me week to week. It felt important that I let her take things at her own pace and for her to have the choice in her hands.

I was aware that for people who have experienced traumatic life events, certain movements can feel exposing or create a sensory recall of an abusive situation. As I taught her the Simple Sleep Sequence, I showed her the movements first, and asked her to tell me if she'd prefer not to do any of the moves, noticing her reactions as I demonstrated each movement; if something looked uncomfortable, I suggested a different movement and checked that with her as well.

When we'd adapted the movements, she came to enjoy the poses, and could feel them releasing tension from her limbs; but if she stayed in a stretch too long or pushed too much, her body would convulse and she would tighten up again. For Tina, it was a process of releasing 'enough but not too much' to create relaxation – slowly, so that her body and mind could trust the release process, with no forcing or straining – and increasing her 'window of tolerance'.

We worked out ways to address Tina's fear of daytime exhaustion. We added some wake-up poses to her morning routine, which she found energising and comforting. She came to enjoy the way she could change how she felt through changing her body, and that she was in control. Then, instead of relying solely on alcohol to calm down and caffeine to pep up, she learned that the stretches and breathwork, after some practice, would work without the side effects. She learned not to overwhelm herself but to work within her window of tolerance, to manage her tension levels throughout the day so they would not build up to unmanageable levels at night.

As she finished her course of our sleep-related sessions, Tina was feeling calmer and more in control, able to get through her days without fear of exhaustion, and she learned how to take a rest in the daytime when she felt tired. The yoga helped her to find a physical sense of safety. As she continued with the stretches and breathing techniques, her level of overall tension lowered, and her ability to work through the things she was afraid of in her therapy sessions improved. For Tina, creating a foundation of bodily safety helped lay the foundation for long-term Sleep Recovery and a growing sense of wholeness.

STEP 5

Release fear, reawaken happy

LIKE MANY CHILDREN OF MY ERA, I read books of myths and fairy tales. If I look back, some of these offered some pretty sinister ideas about what happens to us when we fall asleep. The Greek god of sleep, Hypnos, was the brother of Thanatos, the god of death. Even the immortal Zeus was powerless against Hypnos, who put him to sleep so that other gods could do their will unhindered by Zeus's wishes. The Bible story of Samson holds that the devious Delilah waited until he fell asleep to cut his hair, stealing his power and potency. Sleeping Beauty was punished by being put to sleep for years and years. Being asleep involves vulnerability, and a lack of control. This seems particularly difficult for us, in the modern era.

Dylan Thomas's famous poem about death, 'Do not go gentle into that good night', which was written in 1947, seems to sum up most people's attitude today towards sleep. We appear to be raging against the dying of the light with our high-wattage electric light bulbs, LEDs in every hand, and lights so bright at night they can be seen *far* into space. Perhaps our insomnia is, at least in part, an effect of fighting against darkness and a desire to control our environment.

Darkness can be scary. But in it lies potential, the unknown, and in the case of the human body, the surrender that allows nature to do for us what we cannot do for ourselves through force of will – repair and restore. This is a fundamentally difficult concept to modern people, who have a sense of social and economic mobility and that our worth is determined by what – and how much – we do, earn and accomplish. It is countercultural to want less, do less and truly rest.

If you learn to relax more deeply, look after yourself all day, use all the right tools and practices and still find yourself unable to sleep enough to feel refreshed in the day, it may be time to look at your restlessness more closely: to *hear* what it's saying to you. What is keeping you awake may be trying to wake you up to some deeper truth that is eluding you.

In this step, I explore how insomnia was my own wake-up call, and offer you a couple of simple tools to help you engage more deeply with spiritual aspects of Sleep Recovery. We will look at existential fear, explore joy. We'll end with a call to keep making the changes that have the greatest impact on you and a commitment to waking up happier, remembering that the tools and skills of Sleep Recovery will always be there for you, whenever you need them.

Sleeplessness as a call to awaken

When I was in my 20s, I was always ill, never sleeping, anxious and fearful, I *just* wanted a good night's sleep – and to stop getting sick all the time. The insomnia needed sorting out for any other healing and change to start. Like that canary in the coalmine, my sleep was reporting back from deep down a dark tunnel: something here is toxic. I look at my habits from that time – many of which were somewhat normal for an average American living in a city, just out of university and with an active work and social life – and not only were those habits sabotaging my sleep, but the entire way I viewed my body, energy, emotions, mind and life were deeply misaligned with what is sustainable and healthy. Over the years since then, I have come to view sleep as a part of my life that I safeguard, care for and love. And when my sleep is not happy, it's telling me that *I'm* not happy. Learning to care for my body, mind and emotions has become part of what I would call a 'spiritual' journey.

You see, I was never one who loved to go to sleep. I loved being awake a lot more, reading long into the night after my parents had gone to bed. Back then, we had these plug-in night lights, and I'd put my book under it and the light would fan out on to the pages – at first, of picture books, and then of black-and-white type that would ask me to make the pictures in my head. You might say I was being a naughty kid, not going to bed on time. But even after my mother would soothe me by making circles on my back with her hand, after she'd left and I'd often pop out of bed to read by the night light. It was time for imagination, calm, and other worlds. And even then, I liked time to myself.

But it wasn't until I was 17 that, through a severe trauma, my world fractured and so did my sleep. Between 17 and my mid-20s, I didn't sleep more than three hours at a stretch. I had no idea that what happened would affect me so deeply for so long, because it seemed to me there was an unwritten code for how long it takes to move through the mourning of a death or a loss. I understood so little about what to do when 'existential' questions shake you to your core. Getting to sleep was a process of repairing a compound fracture of every part of myself. And if I can now sleep well, I think it's possible that you can repair your own rest. It may take time and care, but it won't *have to* take you as long as it took me, because we know so much more now.

I have since come to believe that most of us who can't sleep have something that keeps us awake at night. Is it fear, guilt, anger? Something you haven't found a way to lay to rest? If you're sleepless in a soul-aching way, maybe something major has happened in your life that makes you question your place in the world.

Traditional and indigenous medicine models sought to bring a person's entire system back into balance with a combination of plants with healing properties, food and lifestyle changes, *and* spiritual components – of faith, care and love. Back in the day, if you were sick you might have gone to a medicine man or woman, a shaman or a healer who took into account that your *spirit* needed to be involved in your healing. Modern medicine is largely reductionist, focusing on areas of specialism to break the problem down into component parts and resolve ailments at that level. Systemic sleeplessness without a clear physical basis often can't be resolved this way. We can look towards the great mysteries of our humanity to see what's waking us up: existential fears, death anxiety, the stories we've been told, a lack of purpose or fulfilment, a sense of separateness, fragmentation or disconnection, or a longing to know who and what we are at our core.

There were years of bad habits that seemed normal because I lived in a society that taught me to control, command and override my body in order to have the right look, be the right weight, and accomplish the right things. I got the message that being *driven* was a good thing, and I didn't know how to stop. When I couldn't do it – really sort this problem – on my own, I thought: what if what is left is to *undo*. I've since learned that what people refer to as *prayer* is a process of articulating something longed for, and asking for it – from life, nature, a higher power, the divine or God. It felt stronger than an intention, because there was so much power behind it.

This is where a spiritual perspective came in. In order to *undo*, I needed to find, for me, what it was that I was praying to or asking for help. I've since learned that when people need to recover from addictions or life-threatening illnesses, one thing that tends to underpin their way through is tapping into something bigger than their own will or ego – to look to the life-force, nature, or *something* bigger than our individual selves, that heals, and while meditation is a way of slowing down your thoughts, shifting into deeper brainwave patterns and sorting out your mind, the practice of doing it gives you a sense that there is *something* inside, that beyond the hum of thoughts and feelings, in the stillness, there is something essential.

The possibility: sleeplessness as a wake-up call from your soulful self

....

I'm offering you the possibility of seeing your relationship to sleep as one of trusting in the *life force.* Whether you choose to call it your soul or spirit, or something else, your healing involves it. It doesn't matter whether you are an atheist, agnostic, Christian, Muslim, Jewish, Hindu, any other faith or none at all. Yoga, throughout the ages, has been translated as 'union' – not uniting things that are separate, but remembering that we are *actually always whole.* The practices in this book all point in the same direction: a sense of wholeness and developing the *internal* resources that enrich our lives. In this, a kind of soulful or spiritual 'waking up' means we can experience this feeling of fullness, wholeness and connection – through the pleasures and pains, sleepless nights and stressful days as well as in our greatest joys, creative expressions and sweet dreams.

This soulful perspective invites you to look at yourself as a *spiritual* being, connected by a universal life force, or *nature.* I love how the Vietnamese Buddhist teacher Thich Nhat Hanh describes a spiritual dimension in life in a practical way. He says: 'If we have *this capacity*, then we can develop real and lasting spiritual intimacy with ourselves and others...' And that a spiritual dimension to life helps us to feel less afraid: when we bring tenderness to the way we listen to our own human needs, urges and longings, attending to the needs of our bodies, living in alignment with the rhythm of day and night. These form a kind of intimacy that honours the self and our place in the world, and I would call this a spiritual practice.

Spiritual understanding and practice can instil and support in you a sense of trust in nature and in the process of life. It helps to address the fear of death that sits beneath much of our human inability to let go. This can be essential to the process of sleeping well.

When we talk about spirituality, I'm not suggesting a blind belief or dogmatic adherence to a spiritual teaching or concept of the world, but as a soulful *practice* that, as Hanh says, 'brings relief, communication, and transformation'. This seems a very powerful recipe for healing: *relief* – in the form of alleviating tension, pain and agitation; *communication* – in the form of dialogue with symptoms and our habits; and *transformation* – in the form of lasting changes created over time in our bodies, minds and orientation to life itself.

Fear is one of the most powerful forces that can cause us to become sleepless. We have explored the physical, mental and emotional aspects of sleep, all of which fear can affect. For most human beings, fears are a way of relating to something out of balance in life. As we protect ourselves out of fear, this creates physical tension, tightness and shutdown. The sleepless have both *small* fears and colossal, *existential fears*. The smaller *particular fears* are not insignificant, and almost anything can crop up: not being good enough, not being loved, not having enough (money or resources). Part of listening to and working *beyond fear* means being more clearly attuned to what we believe about life and our sense of connection – soulful or spiritual. If we take a soulful or spiritual perspective, we see that the smaller fears can often mask the really big common fears that I call *The Big Three*:

> Not getting something I want
> > Getting something that I don't want
> > > That I will die

There is an old Christian prayer that I learned when I was a child. I've since looked it up. There are several variations, but this is the pithy one I heard from a young age.

> *Now I lay me down to sleep.*
> *I pray the Lord my soul to keep.*
> *If I should die before I wake,*
> *I pray to God my soul to take.*

It's likely that it absolutely terrified me. Who knows: being taught to think about death right before sleep as a child might have contributed to my early insomnia. But fear of death is hardwired into all of us. The primary goal of the human organism is to stay alive, and a fear of death is evolutionarily adaptive. Just the right amount of this fear may prompt us to keep ourselves safe. However, every major religious and spiritual tradition throughout history has sought to explain what happens when we die – giving us comfort, or at least something to believe about what is beyond this life. Many religions even offer instructions for what we can do in order to have a good life after death. Perhaps our modern age has broken these ways of understanding, leaving us without a sense of safety and security, so when we are asked to let go and to turn over our will to nature, to sleep and trust that we will wake, then we can find it deeply distressing.

Getting things we don't want, and not getting what we do want

While taking responsibility for ourselves is a necessary part of being a decent adult, sometimes this can lead us to be wilful – in an unhealthy way. As far as I can tell, life will always involve things outside of our control: we will get things we don't want, and we won't get things we do want. We have to deal with this, and find our way through the best we can; rather than expecting life to be simple, we have to make of it what we will, lest we be dragged under by it all. This, of course, is in the context of not simply slapping ourselves into shape – we must feel the disappointment and move through it (as in Step 4), but once we have allowed the emotions true space and time, there is a possibility that after the storm the weather clears, and our vision opens up once again.

Repairing our sleep requires that we recognise forces greater than our own will and – dare I say it – that we *surrender* to these forces. While this can be somewhat deflating, it can, in fact, be a great relief.

I offer you an exercise that picks up on a point I made in Step 4: it helps to rebalance your ideas about control and surrender, to hand over the big questions in life, to put your concerns *somewhere* in order to let them go. In this I invite you to consider, if you haven't before, how you envision the source of your life. What do you feel is more powerful than your individual ability to control life?

I have heard this principle expressed using all of the words below, by people who range from atheist to devoutly religious. I suggest you choose the one that best fits what you believe, or find a way that expresses it best for you:

Spirit

   Soul

      Source

         Nature

            God

               Universe

                  Life force

                     Higher power

Grant me the serenity to accept the things I cannot change
The courage to change the things I can
And the wisdom to know the difference.

Waking up and finding your spark

In *Man's Search for Meaning*, a small but powerful book that has sold millions of copies since its publication in 1946, Viktor Frankl shares his story of living through the horror of internment in Nazi concentration camps. In his experience, he found a truth: that when our life struggles have meaning, we can *endure*. This doesn't mean that our lives will be easy, without pain, that we won't suffer or that we can control our world. It does mean that when we can find somewhere to put that suffering, some understanding that helps us to move forward with purpose, we can live with more ease. I believe that when we are off course, living with getting-and-spending as our primary goals simply to shore up our sense of security and safety, we know that we are missing something. Many of the people I have treated for insomnia in one-to-one sessions find that once they strip back the first layers of their sleeplessness, they realise there is something soulful in their lives that they have left behind.

For me, when I work as a therapist, there is a frame around each person who sits in the chair or nestles into the sofa. That person has

Serenity for sleep

Try this nightly pre-sleep exercise to practise letting go.
Take out a piece of paper. Write the following questions and leave space for the answers. Give this 5–10 minutes.

- What's bothering me? What am I afraid of, what do I resent, what can't I let go of today?
- What can I change?
- What can't I change?
- Do I need something to help me know which it is?

my full attention – I'm listening carefully not only to what they say and the deeper meaning for them, but I'm also tracking the feeling and the energy behind their words. When talking about a situation: does she light up or does she shrink? Does his voice seem clear and resonant or does it become thin and reedy? Do her eyes sparkle or dim?

There are clear cues to how we feel, and our bodies don't lie. Sometimes, we get so busy, rushed or stressed that we don't know *ourselves* how we feel – and this is where practices like yoga and conscious breathing help tremendously. They help us to cultivate that inner sense of what is happening called *interoception*, which we looked at briefly in Step 1. We can start to track our energy, in terms of our life force and desire, enjoyment and enthusiasm.

> **Enthusiasm** comes from two Greek words – en (to be filled) and Theos (God, or the divine). When we are enthusiastic we are filled with the life force, God, the divine or whatever we call it.
>
> Without enthusiasm for at least some things in life, there is a sense of dryness, a loss of the spark in life. This is one reason that some of my clients find it hard to rest. I believe that on some level the soul (or inner guidance) holds us accountable – that it sometimes doesn't let us rest until we reconnect.

Is there enjoyment and energy in some of the things in life or is every work day a slog to make it to the weekend, or every interaction in the relationship a sacrifice for some later time? Is there a reward so far off in the distance that the day-to-day has become dry and bland? In each person I work with, I look for what they find charming, energising and enjoyable. What is it that you love? What lights you up? And are you spending any of your time bringing that into your life in some way? When we lose this spark, we are diminished overall.

Delaying gratification allows us to control our impulses, pay attention to important tasks, and achieve goals that take time, energy and effort. Most things in life that are worth doing require this of us. We definitely don't need to feel totally gratified all the time. But: if you are mortgaging every present moment for some time in the future when you'll retire, or be happy, or finally have achieved everything you wanted in order to feel you can rest, then you are probably soul-sick – and that could be why you're not sleeping.

If you don't know what lights you up or have forgotten, you may want to re-read this step and ask yourself some questions. Every healing process relies on resourcing. Re-sourcing, if we look at this more deeply, is a coming-back to our source. What can you come back to that brings you joy, happiness, a sense of safety or goodness? What makes you feel whole and light? In order to heal any fractures, you need to actively cultivate your connection to Source.

A final note

....

MY OWN SLEEPLESSNESS was both profoundly painful and a precious gift: I was called to find what was out of balance and learn what I needed to keep connected to my creaturely needs – physical, energetic, mental, emotional and soulful. In the process, creating my own Sleep Recovery and sharing it with others has helped to be of service, which adds to my life's meaning and purpose.

I can also share that the people who have undertaken the Sleep Recovery process in earnest, because they have needed it and have taken this need seriously, have received some great gifts.

Liz got her laugh back. As she kept up her meditation and took time out to rest, she found a sense of amusement and playfulness rounded out what was a fiery, goal-oriented world.

Ollie began putting down roots. Getting into his body began to warm him up, and he started connecting with others, finding a new relationship and more harmony at work.

Cathy realized that although she is in her 'third age' years, the game is far from over. She used the yoga practices to get her spark back, and she's enjoying an acting class that connects her to new people and her creativity.

The yoga poses and practices, and learning that her responses to trauma are both normal and reversible, have helped **Tina** to feel more comfortable in her own skin. She's kept up her yoga and breath work, and begun Somatic Experiencing with a qualified therapist, alongside her long-standing psychotherapy. She's feeling more at ease, and fewer wine bottles make their way into the recycling bin each week. She's flirting with the idea of a 12-step programme to bring the bottle count to zero.

As you've gone through this book, it is my hope that you've found a way to turn your sleeplessness into a positive wake-up call: that you've learned new knowledge, skills and resources that not only assist you with getting to sleep but help you to feel happier, healthier and more fulfilled.

I hope that you will return to this book and integrate what it offers you, so that you can rely on your own internal wisdom- and a deeper sense of safety and soothing. These are always available to you.

Thank you for taking the time to do this: it becomes increasingly important as our world becomes more mechanised and technologised, that we reconnect to our physicality, our sources of inspiration, energy and humanity. This can only help us as we face the personal, environmental and political challenges of our time. It is my hope that by being more human, we become more humane and attuned, not only to ourselves but to each other, and we begin to embody and adopt a more compassionate stance in all we do.

There is a saying that has been attributed to many wise people: be the change that you want to see in the world. When we start to rest easier and wake up happier, perhaps we look after each other with more kindness and compassion.

Acknowledgments

....

GENERAL GRATITUDE

While this work brings together knowledge developed in many fields of study and practice, it also is borne out of tremendous support from colleagues, mentors, friends and family. I don't know if anyone has ever written a book entirely alone. I'm grateful to my sister Diane for showing that writing books is something we Sanfilippo girls *do* and to our parents Margaret and Charles for unflagging support of every kind.

Sleep Recovery was created with the support of friends in my now-hometown of London, UK, but the network of professional and personal support and collegial feedback extends to the US, Greece, Australia, Spain: really all over. They are writers, yogis, therapists, ex-pat family, ad-hoc coaches and purveyors of cups of tea, humour, feedback, and places to stay when needed: Katy Baldock, Amy Beierholm, Katinka Blackford Newman, Beverley Bonner, Lucilla Green, Mark Humphreys-Evans, Theo Kyriakos, Anna Leask, Tamsin Olivier, Chris Plowman, Anais Theyskens, Sivaroshan Sahathevan, Claudia J Smith, Jane de Teliga, Erika Tourell, the late Susan Z. and Rick Watson.

This book is dedicated to Amma, who shows by example that everything given in this life, both the hardships and the gifts, can be offered up in service, and with great love, so that others can, in turn, be of service in *their* own way.

The team at Bloomsbury Green Tree was phenomenal: insightful, patient, reassuring. When I met Charlotte Croft her first questions to me told me that the book we'd make together would be a thing far better than I could have imagined without her. Editor Zoë Blanc was a joy to work with: her understanding, wit and perspective enhanced the book immeasurably. Special thanks to Jenni Davis for copy-editing, and Austin Taylor for design and layout.

Thanks to Masha Pimas' teamwork and perseverance, we have accurate illustrations of the practices which I hope you'll enjoy following at home. Jonathan Thompson, one of my dear students, modelled the male figures in the book with good humour. The talented and hilarious Shaun Levin was a reassuring writing coach, always in the wings when I needed him.

Countless students and clients in workshops, courses, one-to-ones and in the therapy room inspired the amalgamated case studies and asked great questions. I won't name them in order to respect confidentiality, but if we worked together over the years, know that I learned so much in our interactions and that I send you my love and gratitude.

Over the past 15 years, my yoga homes in London have been like the fatherland and the mothership of Sleep Recovery. At Triyoga, Jonathan Sattin and his team have been heroes in making yoga accessible to everyone. Elizabeth Stanley and Lisa Kaley-Isley at Yogacampus and The Life Centre have been champions of yoga therapy and provided support in developing the Sleep Recovery professional training that I now teach in various places around the world. Special thanks go to Heather Mason at the Minded Institute for her support in the early stages of Sleep Recovery's development, as well as her expert input into earlier versions of the training, which involved lectures by Dr Sat Bir Khalsa and Philip Stevens.

Every person who learns yoga has a special place in their heart for their teachers. I've probably had hundreds, but a few must be mentioned in relation to this work. My first, the late Ann Beckerman, gave me the gifts of yoga as poetry and a slow methodical approach – even when I was too young to fully appreciate them. Long before I knew yoga therapy was a *thing*, Anodea Judith, and in particular her work in making the esoteric crystalline and practical, and her ninja-like skill in one-to-one work, inspired me to combine yoga's power with psychotherapy's grounding.

Great appreciation goes to consultant psychiatrist Dr Shivanthi Sathanandan, who offered a practical check of my work, and her support in the development of my previous book, this book, and the Sleep Recovery training.

In large part, Sleep Recovery owes its psyche and soul to transpersonal psychotherapy, a form of therapy that works with – and beyond – the personality to reach into the soul

and spirit. I was taught at the Centre for Counselling and Psychotherapy Education (CCPE) under Nigel Hamilton, Julie Scully, Katy Baldock and Tamsin Olivier. The family of teachers, supervisors and therapists at CCPE helped inform my perspective generally, and particularly my work in Steps 3, 4 and 5. In the UK, you can find low-cost and standard therapy at CCPE in London, often with referrals available across the UK. In the US, the California Institute for Integral Studies (CIIS) is a major hub for training and practice in this area.

In Step 5 and scattered throughout the book is a refrain called the Serenity Prayer, which is used in 12-step addiction recovery programmes.

REFERENCES BY CHAPTER

Sleep Recovery: A new approach

This book is intended to be conversational and inviting for the sleep-deprived, so it leaves out a lot of technical information. If you want more detail, or are a therapist, yoga teacher, healthcare professional or simply curious, you'll find more technical information and detail in my first book, *Yoga Therapy for Insomnia and Sleep Recovery* (London: Singing Dragon, 2019). For a concise overview of mainstream insomnia treatments and details about insomnia and sleep problems from both a clinical and a yoga perspective, please see the chapter I co-authored with Dr. Khalsa in Heather Mason and Kelly Birch's *Yoga for Mental Health* (Pencaitland: Handspring, 2018).

In framing the sleep types, I'm indebted to my local Ayurvedic colleagues Jono Condous and Xenia Bolomiti who brought this wisdom to life for me, and to Marc Holzman for his encouragement. Works by Dr Vasant Lad and Mark Frawley have served as references and expanded the perspectives threaded through this book.

While this book draws its steps from an interpretation of the five layers (*koshas*) as outlined in one of the yoga traditions, many of the concepts in the latter chapters are influenced by friends, colleagues and collaborators with experience and knowledge drawn from 12-step fellowships devoted to recovering from substance and process addictions as a structured return to wholeness. Where sleep problems are associated with addictions (to drugs, alcohol, sex or gambling) or compulsive activities like overeating, anorexia, codependency or debt, these free anonymous programmes can provide a vital companion to Sleep Recovery.

Step 1: Repair your body

Two classic books on sleep hygiene and holistic views of insomnia informed Sleep Recovery from its early days: Gregg Jacobs' *Say Goodnight to Insomnia* (Emmaus: Rodale, 2009), and Peter Hauri and Shirley Linde's *No More Sleepless Nights* (San Francisco: Jossey-Bass, 1996). An overview of insomnia as a condition can be found in article from 2013 simply called 'Insomnia' by D.J. Buysse, in the *Journal of the American Medical Association* (309(7): 706–716).

For information about yoga postures, the classic *Light on Yoga* by B.K.S. Iyengar, first published by George Allen & Unwin in 1966, was an early resource for me: straightforward and comprehensive. More contemporary books are plentiful. To understand yoga more generally, Georg Feuerstein's books offer some grounding. *The Path*

of Yoga: An Essential Guide to Its Principles and Practices (Boulder: Shambhala, 1996) puts yoga into its context and *The Psychology of Yoga: Integrating Eastern and Western Approaches for Understanding the Mind* (Boulder: Shambhala, 2014) points to the intersection of yoga and psychology.

The chart in this book on the caffeine content of common beverages draws heavily upon the Caffeine Informer website, by kind permission. McGill University in Canada maintains a site that explains the brain and the effects of caffeine and GABA among other things: thebrain.mcgill.ca. I drew upon this resource in checking several sections of this book. There are many studies on sleep and shift work. The main one I have referred to is: D.B. Boivin, P. et al.'s 2012 paper, 'Photic resetting in night-shift work: impact on nurses' sleep', published in *Chronobiology International* (29(5): 619-28). The Mayo Clinic in the US has information on light therapy for Seasonal Affective Disorder (SAD) on its website: mayoclinic.org.

Step 2: Replenish your energy

In this step, I refer to the following books: *The Relaxation Response* by Herbert Benson with Miriam Z. Klipper (Glasgow: Avon, 2000); and *The Healing Power of the Breath: Simple Techniques to Reduce Stress and Anxiety, Enhance Concentration, and Balance Your Emotions* by Richard P. Brown and Patricia L. Gerbarg, (Boulder: Shambhala, 2012). The restorative poses in this chapter were adapted through my personal practice from *Relax and Renew: Restful Yoga for Stressful Times*. This book was originally published in 1995 by the queen of restorative yoga, physiotherapist and yoga teacher Judith Hanson Lasater.

I also drew on an article aimed at yoga therapists 'Mechanisms of pranayama: how respiratory physiology can refine your teaching' by Heather Mason in *Yoga Therapy Today* (International Association of Yoga Teachers, Spring edition, 2017). The Breath of Joy is a modified version of Amy Weintraub's practice found in *Yoga for Depression* (New York: Broadway Books, 2004).

If you're interested in yoga breathing in greater depth, the classic is *Light on Pranayama* by BKS Iyengar (London: HarperCollins, 1981), and later books like *The Breathing Book* by Donna Farhi (New York: Henry Holt, 1996), and *Breathe* by Jean Hall (London: Quadrille, 2016) provide accessible modern takes on yoga breathing.

The Kundalini yoga breathing in this chapter is also outlined in Dr Sat Bir Singh Khalsa's research, and featured in a Harvard Health book you can find online called *Your Brain On Yoga*: harvardhealthbooks.org.

The 4:7:8 breath in this chapter was popularised by the American medical wellbeing expert Dr Andrew Weil, and a description can be found on his web site, drweil.com, if you search Relaxing Breath or 4-7-8 Breath.

Step 3: Reclaim your mind

Thanks go to Jillian Lavender and Michael Miller of the London Meditation Centre and the New York Meditation centre, for teaching me Vedic meditation, a latter development on from Transcendental meditation. I recommend Sally Kempton's book *Meditation for the Love of It* (Boulder: Sounds True, 2011) and credit my

teacher and colleague Carlos Pomeda for his demonstration of the power of presence of the teacher in meditation. The meditation that focuses on the sensation of breath in the nose is practised in some traditions of Vipassana meditation, which is offered at many centres worldwide, often on a by-donation basis.

Jon Kabat-Zinn is the most widely known proponent of mindfulness in the west. He has many resources including *Wherever You Go, There You Are* (New York: Hyperion, 2004). I also drew on Dr. Barbara Mariposa's *Mindfulness Playbook: How to Bring Calm and Happiness into Your Daily Life* (London: Hodder and Stoughton, 2016).

For information about cognitive behavioural therapy (CBT), please refer to the websites of the NHS in the UK, and the National Institute of Health in the US. As CBT is a very structured form of psychotherapy, it lends itself to research easily and is therefore among the most well-documented of psychotherapeutic interventions.

Step 4: Restore a sense of calm

In this step we deal with emotions. You can find further resources on emotions in a variety of places. One resource is the interactive tool The Atlas of Emotions, created by Paul and Eve Ekman with support from the Dalai Lama (atlasofemotions.org/). The emotional release technique on page 154 is adapted from a practice taught by Thich Nat Hahn. There are many other books and resources in the worlds of Buddhism, psychology and psychotherapy that can prove invaluable in understanding and navigating the difficult emotions that can sabotage our sleep.

I also referred to non-violent

communication (NVC) in this step, which was pioneered by Marshall Rosenberg. His book *Nonviolent Communication: A Language of Life* (Encinitas: PuddleDancer, 2015) is a good place to turn, if interpersonal conflict and having difficult conversations keeps you up at night.

The drama triangle I refer to in this chapter is a way to understand the dynamics of interpersonal relationships and conflict developed by Dr Stephen Karpman as a student of Eric Berne, M.D., who is often referred to as the father of a branch of psychotherapy called Transactional Analysis. I refer to this in Steps 3 and 4 as it relates to our thoughts and our emotions.

The work on post-traumatic insomnia in Step 4 benefitted greatly from my personal work with and advice from Frances Ross, an early student of Dr Peter Levine. Pages 166–7 summarise trauma-related concepts that you'll find in books by Dr. Levine. His classic *Waking the Tiger: Healing Trauma* (Berkeley: North Atlantic Books, 1997) and the more recent *Healing Trauma: A Pioneering Program for Restoring the Wisdom of Your Body* (Boulder: Sounds True, 2008) are good places to turn, as is *In an Unspoken Voice: How the Body Releases Trauma and Restores Goodness* (Berkeley: North Atlantic Books, 2010). There is also a growing body of literature on the links between trauma and addiction. The work of Dr Gabor Maté and others are useful if this chapter resonates with you and you want to know more.

A short training with Alexandra Cat, the London-based adjunct of the Trauma Centre in Boston, introduced me to David Emerson's work on trauma-sensitive yoga, which also informed this section. For more information and detail, you can read David Emerson's book *Trauma-Sensitive Yoga in Therapy: Bringing the Body into Treatment* (New York: W. W. Norton and Company, 2015) and Dagmar Härle's *Trauma-Sensitive Yoga* (London: Singing Dragon, 2017).

Thanks in this area go to Linda Karle and Theodora Wildcroft for comments on earlier drafts.

Step 5: Release fear, reawaken happy

For the fifth step, I drew upon many spiritual traditions and turned to people I felt offered us some practical wisdom. What would people far wiser than I say about what's keeping us awake? Because the spiritual and soulful aspect of life can feel elusive, day to day language can be thin on the ground. Thich Nhat Hahn's book *How to Love* (London: Rider, 2016) fell into my lap when I was writing this chapter, and his words are reflected therein.

If you are feeling lost and want a gentle nudge towards being who you are more fully, *The Soul's Code* by James Hillman (New York: Random House, 1996) offers some loving words that might help with the search for your calling.

For those seeking help beyond these pages, it's my intention that you will see more qualified Sleep Recovery practitioners spring up throughout the world, and new resources will be created in the coming years. Stay tuned!

www.sleeprecoveryyoga.com

Index